BEYOND THE CHAIR

Betté Pratt

To order additional copies of this book, contact:
Bookwhip
1-855-339-3589
www.bookwhip.com

This book is dedicated to my aunt.
Sara inspired everyone she met to look beyond
her chair to her Lord.
I still have several of her paintings and also play the piano
because of her inspiration.
I know if she lived in this day and age she would have been married
to someone who would not have let her chair come between them.

—Betté Pratt

PROLOGUE

Colleen turned on her call light and waited… and waited.

"Why don't they answer? I'll wet the bed if they don't answer soon," she mumbled.

Several more minutes passed before a tiny voice over the intercom said, "Yes, Mrs. Bernard, do you need something?"

"You know they told me to call for help the first time I needed to get up to the bathroom! Send somebody right away!" Colleen said, urgently.

"I'll be right there." The light went off and Colleen waited… Finally, a nurse aid came in and said with a smile, "You need to go to the restroom, Mrs. Bernard? I've come to help you."

Colleen sat up in the bed and swung her legs over the edge. She felt perfectly fine and put her feet down, ready to stand on them. The nurse reached over and took her arm to steady her, but didn't pull her to her feet. Colleen made it to a standing position then took a step. Finally, she was on her way for that all important first trip to the bathroom. However, the ten feet to the tiny restroom in the corner of her room seemed like it was at least a mile long. She sighed when she collapsed onto the seat.

After she washed her hands, the girl still stood outside the door, so Colleen asked, "What took you so long to answer my call? I nearly had an accident, you know."

Instantly uncomfortable, the young woman looked down at the floor. Finally, she said, "Umm, none of us were at the desk when your light came on. Something happened in the nursery and we were all in there."

"In the nursery! What happened?"

"I…ah…think the head nurse'll be in to talk with you soon."

Colleen made it back to her bed in record time under her own steam and the nurse aid fled from the room. Colleen laid her head back on the pillow and looked up at the ceiling. The TV was blaring and disgustedly she hit the remote to silence the beast. When she came in last night in labor she was the only one, her baby, Sandra Candice Bernard, was the only baby in the nursery. Perhaps while she slept this morning another woman had come in and given birth so that there were two babies in the nursery now.

What could have happened in the nursery?

From the way the girl had talked, someone would be in right away, but no one came to talk with her, as the woman had indicated. Colleen lay in the bed and fussed and fumed. Nearly half an hour later a different nurse wheeled the bassinet in for Colleen to feed her baby. Tiny Sandy was letting everyone know she was hungry, but she was bundled up in her pink blanket and pink knitted cap. Colleen knew she couldn't be cold, especially as warm as it was.

Colleen eagerly reached for Sandy. The baby had weighed only six and a half pounds, but she was perfect, beautiful. Her hair was dark, just like hers and Charlie's but with some curls in it. Her eyes were blue, neither she nor Charlie had blue eyes, but it didn't matter, Sandy was their first baby, somewhere in their family had to be someone with blue eyes. Besides, didn't baby's eyes change color?

The nursery worker made sure Colleen and Sandy were comfortable together then she left, pulling the door nearly closed. Instantly, Colleen was lost in her baby and forgot about what the first nurse said. Before the nurse came back for Sandy, Charlie came in and sat on the bed beside Colleen. He slid his arm behind her and looked tenderly at his child. When Sandy didn't suck anymore, Colleen took her from her breast, but she looked solemnly at her mommy and daddy. Colleen slid her hand under her neck to support her head and under her bottom to hold her. Sandy's legs didn't curl up, but fell over Colleen's wrist both she and Charlie noticed it.

Charlie was about to push the call button when two nurses walked in the room and right behind them the Bernard's doctor. Colleen scowled and Charlie looked from one to the other and asked, "What do we owe all this notoriety to?"

Both nurses stepped back and reluctantly the doctor stepped forward. Nervously, he wiped his hand over his mouth and cleared his throat. The man swallowed, but even so the first word came out in a squeak. "Mr. and Mrs. Bernard, Charlie and Colleen, umm, there was an accident in the nursery very early today. Umm, when the night nurse was changing her diaper, umm, the baby slipped from her hands and fell on the edge of the changing table." The doctor dropped his eyes to the floor, his voice also dropped to nearly a whisper, "We think perhaps the baby sustained some spinal cord injury, she's not moving her legs as she was before."

Charlie came off the bed and in one huge step his six foot frame loomed in front of the doctor. Both nurses stepped back, as the foreboding figure looked from the doctor to each woman. "You're telling me our baby is crippled now?" His voice boomed out, those huddled around the call system at the desk were nearly blasted from the box.

"I...I wouldn't say that, Charlie," the doctor stuttered, "but we do need a neurologist to make an evaluation before she leaves the hospital."

"Well, be about it!" he demanded.

"Yes! Yes, I'll get right on that!" Both he and the two nurses fled, Charlie watched in stunned silence before he turned back to his wife. The door stood wide open, the staff had fled too quickly to close it.

Colleen clutched the baby close to her heart. Sandy finally had shut her eyes. Her fists held some of her mommy's hair, but her legs drooped unless Colleen put her arm under them. Silent tears slid down her cheeks as the words the doctor told them began to sink in. She looked down at the sleeping baby. She was a beautiful child, now that she was passed the first day of life her cheeks were rosy and if her eyes were open they sparkled with intelligence. Colleen felt the tiny legs hang against her arm and guessed there wasn't any pain, she hadn't cried since she started nursing, but how could the baby sleep so peacefully?

However, there was pain in Colleen's heart. Their baby, their perfect, beautiful, first born baby wasn't perfect any more.

Three months later

"But Charlie," Colleen whispered, as they both looked down at the sleeping baby lying in her crib. "The doctor said we'll have to wait until she gets a little older before they can truly tell the damage and how permanent it is."

Fiercely, Charlie said, "Yes, I know that's what he said, but I still say we should take her to the church elders and have them pray over her. She shouldn't be a cripple the rest of her life! God can't let this happen to her! Doesn't it say somewhere that the elders should pray and the person would be healed?"

"Yes, Charlie, that's in James. It says,

> 'Is any one of you sick? He should call for the elders of the church to pray over him and anoint him with oil in the name of the Lord. And the prayer offered in faith will make the sick person well; the Lord will raise him up. If he has sinned, he will be forgiven.' (James 5:14,15)

But do you think this…?"

"Of course! I'll call the pastor and see when they can come."

A few days later, their pastor and three deacons from their church came to the house. Charlie let them in, while Colleen went for the baby. In preparation for this event, Sandy was dressed in a lovely infant outfit. Colleen brought the sleeping child from her bed in the nursery to the living room. All the men crowded around her to see the baby close up, but none of them touched her. The four church men were all older than Charlie and Colleen and had children of their own, but it was easy to see that Sandy was different. No matter how Colleen held her, her legs didn't move on their own.

After Colleen settled in a chair, Pastor Stanley uncomfortably looked across the room and said, "Umm, well, Charlie, come hold your baby and let's put that oil on her and pray. We should see those legs curl up in only minutes."

Charlie scowled. "What's wrong with Colleen holding her and I stand with them, Pastor? I think it should be all three of us."

The man licked his lips, looked from one of his deacons to the other. They in turn wouldn't look at anything but the floor. Pastor Stanley swallowed and finally nodded. "Yeah, sure, that's a good idea. It should be a united thing here. Umm, we'll gather around you when the three of you're ready."

Charlie came to his wife and helped her stand, then slid his arms around her, putting them under his baby. "Okay, here we are, Pastor. You have that oil you promised you'd bring?"

Reaching into his pocket, he said, "Yes, the bottle's right here in my pocket. Come on, men, gather 'round so there's no gap in this circle." The men shuffled closer, their heads bowed and acting very uncomfortable. They did as the pastor asked and stood shoulder to shoulder between Charlie and the pastor. Pastor Stanley pulled out a small bottle from his pocket, uncorked it and let a drop fall on Sandy's forehead. Still holding the bottle in one hand, he placed the other on Sandy's head. "Come on, men, touch her somewhere."

Reluctantly, the three men did as the pastor asked. Now there were four large hands covering Sandy's body. Everyone bowed his head and Pastor Stanley said, "Father, God, Charlie and Colleen have this little tyke and she's not, umm, got the use of her legs. We're praying you'll touch her body and, umm, heal her so's she's good as new. Umm, we ask this in Jesus name, Amen."

Colleen opened her eyes of course, they were on her baby snug in her arms. The drop of oil still pooled and glistened on her forehead. The baby's hands had relaxed as she fell more deeply asleep, but her legs still hung down on Colleen's arm. Colleen raised her head and looked at the silver heads of the men around her. They were also looking at the baby.

Pastor Stanley took his hand away, so the other men did, too. He glanced up at Colleen. "Wake her up, she's really sound asleep."

Colleen gently lifted the baby to her shoulder and patted her on the back. Sandy let out a burp and looked up at her daddy and smiled. She raised her hands, wanting him to hold her, so Charlie picked her off Colleen's shoulder. However, her legs still hung limp from her body, they didn't move at all. Without a word, Charlie looked at Pastor Stanley.

The older man licked his lips. Looked again at the baby's unmoving legs. Obviously Sandy's condition hadn't changed. At a loss, Pastor Stanley cleared his throat and said, "Well, I guess you folks didn't have enough faith, the Lord didn't heal her."

Charlie hugged his baby to his chest. He glared at the man, covered Sandy's ears and bellowed, "OUT!! Get out!! All of you get out!"

The men turned and fled the room. Charlie, holding his baby close, followed them to the front door. Pastor Stanley yanked it open and the four older men fled. Charlie watched as they ran to the car and slammed the door behind them. Colleen still stood in the center of the room tears were streaming down her cheeks and her empty arms hanging at her sides.

ONE

Twenty-five years later

It was spring in Georgia, but of course, in the mountains of northern Georgia not all the snow had melted off the highest peaks. However, Ramon was swamped with requests for his services as a guide in those mountains. He'd been running a one man operation for three years, but his fame had finally catapulted him into a man in demand.

Looking at his appointment book, just as the phone started ringing again, he sighed, "I am going to have to hire someone to take phone calls and keep me squared away. I've double booked again, I'll have to call that one and reschedule."

He picked up the phone after the third ring and said, "DeLord's Hiking and Camping Services, this is Ramon. How can I help you?"

"Mr. DeLord, this is Jason Harris, my wife and I and three children have decided on a back-to-nature vacation this year. We haven't made any firm plans on dates, I'm pretty flexible on that, but sometime after school lets out. Could we arrange something like that with you?"

Paging through his book to July's calendar, Ramon said, "Yes, Mr. Harris, I have the week of July seventeenth open. Would that work for you?"

"Yes, that's a Sunday, though, couldn't we come on Saturday?"

"I'm sorry, I have one group coming back on the sixteenth, I couldn't get ready to leave again before the next morning at the earliest, and that hinges on you folks having everything ready and packed for travel. Can that be done, could you folks handle that?"

"Yes, the children are teenagers and we've camped and hiked before, we'll have everything together, but we've never hiked in your area before, so we would need a guide. Yes, the seventeenth would work for us. That would give us Saturday to close up and load up here and drive there. Could we come back the next Saturday?"

"That would work perfectly for me, Mr. Harris. I've written your name in my appointment book and it's all set. Thanks for calling and using DeLord's."

"Thank you! We're looking forward to it already."

Ramon replaced the receiver with another sigh. Paging back through the book he realized he was booked solid starting next Friday all the way through July twenty-third as of that phone call, with only a day or two scattered throughout those months when he could be back to take more appointments. He knew as soon as he put a pack on his back that he missed some possible bookings. Since his operation was so seasonal, he needed to stay busy every possible day during the seven months when the weather was warm enough for hiking and camping.

He picked up one of the camping and hiking magazines he subscribed to and found an ad for the same thing he did here in Georgia, only that place was in New Mexico. "Well," he muttered, "I have just as many beautiful scenes here as that picture. I'll make up an ad, send it in and see what becomes of it. Maybe next year I can hire another guide."

He began writing down an ad similar to the one in the magazine, but the phone rang again. He shook his head and picked up the receiver.

Leafing through a colorful magazine Ed, Sandy's brother, subscribed to, Sandy exclaimed, "Mom, look at this ad! Look at the absolutely beautiful scenery as a background! I think I'll make out this application and see if I can get this job. It calls for someone with artistic ability and I'm dying to do some painting in a place besides the Schuylkill River Waterway. I'm tired of trying to make the same scenery look different."

"But Sandy!" Colleen exclaimed, "You'd have to move away! Sandy, how could you do that?" Sandy saw the unspoken words *'to me'* written on her face. "Why…"

After a long sigh, Sandy said, "Yes, Mom, I would have to move away. I am twenty-five years old, you know. I know how to cook, clean, dress and move myself from point 'A' to point 'B'. What are you trying to protect me from?"

"But you've never lived anywhere but here!" Colleen exclaimed, nearly hysterical.

"I know that. I also know Daddy has built a ramp from the back door down to the driveway. I can get from there to any car that I want. This afternoon I have an appointment with the driving school." Sandy raised her hand to keep Colleen from talking, she'd opened her mouth, but Sandy continued, "Someone there put me in touch with a company who will rent me a van with a lift. There's a rent to own option that I'm pretty sure I can handle. As soon as it comes in, I'll put the lessons I've had to learn to drive to use. You, Daddy and Edwin are much too busy to always be available to cart me around and Marcy's out of the question, of course."

Tears pooled in Colleen's eyes. "But Sandy… What about…?" She gestured at the metal object that held Sandy's body.

Exasperated, Sandy exclaimed, "Mom, stop! So I'm in a wheelchair who cares! It doesn't bother me, why should it bother you?"

Colleen turned away. She and Charlie had often talked about how independent their oldest child was or wanted to be. Charlie had warned her over and over that Sandy didn't like how her mom hovered over her and tried to pamper her, especially since she'd turned twenty-five last December. Ever since Sandy had been old enough to talk and move herself in her own wheelchair, she had been pushing her mom away.

Moments later, Sandy picked up the phone after one ring and the voice said, "Miss Bernard, we received notice today that your van came in last evening. We'll send your instructor by your place so you can go with him to pick it up. What time today would work for you?"

Instantly excited, Sandy exclaimed, "Any time! I knew it would be in some day this week, so I've only tentatively scheduled in my week. Send him around any time he's available."

"How's eleven o'clock, will that work?"

"Great! I'll be waiting."

Of course, Colleen was hovering in the kitchen as Sandy hung up the phone. Unshed tears glistened in her eyes, as she said, "Honey that was about the van?"

"Yes Mom. It came in last night. My instructor is coming for me at eleven so we can go pick it up and I can have my first chance behind the wheel."

"So I'll be by at one o'clock to pick you up from the school."

"No, Mom, that won't be necessary. I've driven a simulator at the school and been out with my instructor in a van that they have, twice. I feel very confident that I'll be driving my van home after we pick it up."

Without a word, Colleen turned back and stuck her hands in her dishwater, even though there were no dishes and the water was nearly cold. Tears slid down her cheeks and plopped into the water. No matter what she did, her daughter was determined to make her own way in spite of the road blocks thrown up in front of her. Before Colleen could control herself enough to speak, Sandy wheeled from the kitchen back to her conservatory.

The girl was talented there was no question about that. She'd had only a year of piano lessons, but she played so proficiently that her teacher had dismissed her. She and her brother had rigged up a device for the sustaining pedal so she could use it without the use of her feet, but not so a normal person couldn't use the pedal on the piano. Now she gave lessons to the neighborhood children. Her first pupil, whom she graduated five years ago, now played professionally for the city symphony orchestra.

Not only that, between her school lessons, which Colleen had taught, Sandy had started at a pre-school age to draw and paint. At first, she had taken picture postcards and copied them onto drawing paper. It wasn't long before she'd grabbed snapshots her dad took and put the enlarged scenes onto her papers. Several years ago she'd switched to oils and water colors and last spring she'd had her second gallery showing in the library downtown. She'd sold every one. Everyone knew she could make a living just with her paintings.

Colleen listened as Sandy lost herself in her music. She shook her head, if only God had healed her or seen fit to let the neurosurgeons fix her when she was a baby, she could be a world renowned pianist by now. Instead, she sat in that awful chair, with legs that were useless and unnatural looking and played her heart out. Not only that, now she was getting a van that she could use all by herself. It had a lift which she could operate, either from the inside or outside and there was no seat behind the steering wheel. All the controls were on the dash or within arm's reach so she could drive it. Colleen sniffed and took her wet hands from the water. The water from her hands now mingled with the tears coming from her eyes. Charlie would tell her to let her go, to take her hands off, but this was her first born they were talking about!

Ramon was back from a three day backpacking trip with a church group from Atlanta. He'd washed clothes and repacked his backpack for tomorrow's group. Now he sat in his office chair, he'd answered the last voicemail message and now he was booked until Labor Day. He'd picked up the mail that the post office saved for him until he came in for it. He'd had a mail basket full when he went for it this morning. They were good enough to spare him the junk mail, so he only had his bills and other important letters to sift through when he got down to it. He set the bills to one side and picked up a letter with a return address from Philadelphia. He rarely received mail from a big city so far away. Quickly he slit it open and pulled out an application.

"Ah, my first answer to the ad I placed!"

The first line read: <u>Sandra C. Bernard</u> it was dated <u>June 3</u>. Had he been gone a *month* without checking his mail? He checked other letters in his pile, this was the oldest, but there were others dated right around that time. Surely he'd been back, in and out since the third! He read on. Sandra was applying for the job he'd posted in the magazine. He'd placed the ad to run for two months, May and June. If he couldn't get a receptionist in that time, he'd have to ask his cousin to help out. Well, she wasn't really a cousin, but he thought of her like a cousin. He shook his head, he didn't really want her for the job.

Ramon finished reading the application, set it aside and opened other letters. No other correspondence was about the job he'd offered. He was a bit disappointed he'd wished for a little competition. That made him grin. He set everything in an appropriate pile and, since his stomach reminded him that breakfast had been only coffee and a granola bar, he'd better put something in it. He trotted to the kitchen and made a sandwich, a double decker, took a huge bite then made another, put them on a plate and went back to his desk. He'd call this Sandra Bernard. It couldn't hurt to call.

The phone rang, he waited through another two rings until a woman's breathless voice said, "Hello, this is Bernard's."

The lady sounded like an older woman that was probably good. "May I speak with Sandra Bernard, please? This is Ramon DeLord calling."

"She's not here right now. This is her mother, could I take a message?"

"Yes, I'm calling in reference to an ad she answered. I'll give you my number, when could she call me back? Unfortunately, I'll only be here today."

"I'll… I'll have her call you later, perhaps this evening?"

"Yes, that's fine, as long as it's today."

Sandy's heart sounded like her piano playing without the pouch, like a jackhammer in her chest as she drove her instructor's van to the dealer. Finally, she would get her own van! Ed got his own wheels when he was twenty. He'd worked all summer and saved every cent for the old clunker. Of course, she didn't have that luxury, she had to have money up front for a down on a new van that was wheelchair equipped and those, she discovered, cost the stratosphere.

At the dealer, the instructor opened his door and stepped out, then operated the lift so Sandy could get out. She was ready, anxious to see her van and get behind the wheel. Minutes later, she was on the pavement and waited as the instructor raised the lift to its traveling position. She operated her electric chair next to her instructor, on their way toward the showroom.

A smiling salesman left the showroom as they approached. "You are Sandra Bernard?" the man looked at her instructor.

Sandy smiled and said, "Yes! I'm Sandy I understand my van's here?"

The man nodded, but continued to look at the instructor. "This van has a wheelchair lift." He then asked, "Ahh, how will you get both vans from here? Is someone else in your van?"

Sandy, being the, in-your-face-no-nonsense person that she was, wheeled herself between the salesman and her instructor. Before the man could answer the salesman, she said, "Mister, I told you I'm Sandy Bernard! I came to collect my van. I paid the down and the first three months. My instructor will go with me on a test run then I'll bring him back for his van. Do I make myself clear?"

The salesman finally looked at Sandy and mumbled, "Ah, yes, ma'am, I guess you have. I'm sorry for the slight."

Her words curt, she said, "Thank you. Where is the van?"

"It's... ah... over here. I'll get the keys right away." The last few words came back to them on the breeze as the man escaped.

"I'd appreciate that!" Sandy watched the man run away.

When the salesman was out of sight, Sandy turned to her instructor, her eyes blazing. "Why do people do that?" she exclaimed. "Is it because I'm sitting and they assume I'm not an adult or I'm dim-witted?"

The instructor looked down at the very intelligent young woman and shook his head. "I'm afraid it's one or both of those, Sandy. Sometimes they even raise their voices, acting as if the handicapped person is also deaf."

"I know! I've had that happen to me, too."

The man came back with keys dangling from his fingers. He pasted on that huge smile many car salesmen wear when they're trying to make a sale. Holding them almost out of Sandy's reach, he said reluctantly. "Here you are!"

Still not happy, Sandy grabbed the keys. "Thank you! We parked over there, so that van shouldn't be in your way. We'll take a run in this and be back before a half hour's over. Everything's signed, isn't it?"

"Yes, Ma'am. I checked when I went back for the keys. Everything's in order. I guess you went over with our ordering manager what to expect on the van."

"Yes, I did." She gave the man barely a nod and whirled the chair around. Heading in the direction the man had pointed, she said, "Thanks, we'll be back."

The instructor followed, but he knew Sandy wanted to do everything for herself, since this was now her van and she must work with it to her own satisfaction each time she went somewhere. He watched her insert the key in the side of the van, then watched as the large passenger door opened. The salesman went with the instructor, but neither spoke, since they were intent on watching Sandy. Perhaps the salesman was worried about the merchandise that was still on his lot.

As she and the dealer owner had worked out, there were two key locks on the side of the van. The first one opened the large sliding door. A second key in the second lock worked the lift mechanism, unfolded it and brought it to the ground. Without looking at the men, she wheeled herself to the lift and propelled herself onto it, then pushed the button on the handle for it to leave the ground. When she was inside the van she used the controls inside that brought the lift into the van and closed the door. There were seats in the van for passengers, but there was a large open area for her to reach the driver's spot. She wheeled herself into the driver's spot and anchored the chair in place.

The salesman stood and watched even after Sandy had closed the big door, but the instructor opened the passenger door, slid onto the seat and closed the door. By now, Sandy had the chair locked behind the wheel and had inserted the proper key into the ignition. "Finally," she sighed. "I guess that man didn't think I could do all that without him watching."

Sandy put the stick in gear and her instructor said, "Apparently not. He probably doesn't have much dealing with handicapped people. Did it work okay for you?"

"Perfect. I felt no hesitation anywhere. Let's get out of here! I don't like an audience."

Sandy maneuvered the city streets close to the dealership very well and soon felt comfortable behind the wheel of her new van. As her instructor praised her, she drove back to the dealership parking lot and since everything was taken care of, she stopped beside the instructor's van and he got out. She waved there was no reason for her to stay until he had placed the driver's seat in position so he could drive away.

Colleen reluctantly replaced the receiver back on the wall hangar. She didn't want Sandy going to Georgia for a job. What was wrong with staying here, drawing and painting scenes along the Schuylkill River? She had her piano students, besides their weekly payments and the money she made from her frequent gallery showings, she made good money. She even had a market for her hand crafts. Why did she want to go way far away to Georgia for a job?

She'd written the number and the man's name very small on a small piece of paper. She picked it up and put it under Sandy's napkin at her place at the table. Maybe she wouldn't see it and wouldn't call tonight. The man said he'd be gone tomorrow, maybe she wouldn't find it until breakfast and that would be too late. Colleen sighed, she could only hope.

Only a few minutes later, Colleen looked out the kitchen window to see a light blue van come to a stop outside. She scowled, but then a minute later, the back passenger door slowly opened. Colleen's heart skittered into her throat and she ran for the back door. However, before she could get down the ramp, the lift was extending and then stopped. Colleen heart lodged in her throat as she watched Sandy propel her wheelchair onto it and lowered herself to the ground. Colleen stood like a statue.

"Mom! Isn't this perfectly awesome? I'm so thrilled! This thing works like a charm." Still on the lift, she looked up to the back porch. "You want to come for a ride? I'd love to take you and show this off."

No, I don't want to go for a ride! She wanted her little girl back again. She wanted to take care of her, to love her and shield her from all those nasty people who look down their noses on cripples. She licked her lips and said, "I'll get my purse."

9

Only a few minutes after they left, Charlie drove up on the driveway, pushed the garage door opener for his slot and drove in. He went to the back door and scowled when it was locked. Colleen's car was still in her spot, why wasn't she at home? Had one of her sisters come by and taken her and Sandy shopping? He hadn't heard anything mentioned about a trip to town over breakfast, but at six o'clock, Colleen wasn't much for talking.

He set his lunch pail on the counter and went in the bedroom to change clothes. He needed to get downstairs to his workshop to finish that commission piece. In two days the lady from down the street would come for the doll's highchair he'd made for her daughter's birthday. One more coat of finish would do it and it had to be very, very dry before she could have it.

Charlie had just pulled the door to the basement open when the light blue van pulled up outside the kitchen windows. The horn tooted, he scowled and headed for the back door. Colleen was getting out when he arrived on the back porch. She looked up at him and said, "Honey, Sandy wants to take you for a ride around the block." She reached back for her purse.

"That's her new van? Terrific!"

"Umm, yes."

He strode down the ramp in four long strides and slid in while Colleen stepped back. A grinning young woman said, "Dad, what do you think?"

Charlie slammed the door and thumped the dash. "Girl, this is fabulous! I'm so proud of you! So your mother let you take her for a ride?"

Sandy put the stick in reverse and moved slowly down the driveway and stopped at the street, before she said, "Yeah. I was shocked, too. Of course, she held onto that armrest over there the whole time, but she didn't gasp or anything."

Charlie chuckled. "I'm amazed."

"Yeah, now if I can hear from that job I applied for, I'll be happy as a clam."

Growing serious, Charlie asked, "You don't think someone's called about it and your mom took the message and hid it, do you?"

Sandy swiped at her eye and glanced at her dad. "Do you really think she'd do that, Dad? I know she doesn't want me to go away, but surely she wouldn't be that devious, would she?"

"Honey, I don't know. I should hope not."

They had turned a corner, so were out of sight of their home. Sandy pulled over to the side of the street and put the stick in park. Still with a tear hanging on an eyelash, she turned to her dad and said, "Daddy, will you pray about it? Really, I hate to hurt Mom, but if I don't go away she will be forever babying and pampering me. She doesn't do that to Ed or Marcy. You know how much I want to be me."

Charlie reached across from the passenger seat and laid his hand on her arm that was resting on the control arm of her chair. Sandy turned her hand over and fit her hand into her dad's, as he said, "I know, Honey, yes, lets pray right now. Our Father in heaven, we want to thank You for giving us life, we love You for that. Lord, we know You love us, because You sent Your Son to be our Substitute, to give His life to take away our sins. Sandy is here at the threshold of a life-changing situation. She has sent an application for a job that will be out of town. You know her mother wants to keep her here so she can pamper her and keep her hidden from life. It has been some time since Sandy has sent this information and she has not heard from it. Please, Father, don't let this be because her mother has hidden or destroyed it. We pray in Jesus Name, Amen."

"Amen. Thanks, Dad," Sandy sighed and started up again.

Ramon finished writing his checks and looked at the last total. He sighed, he was doing all right by himself, but if that Sandra called back and took a job with him, how would he pay her? He didn't have much in the way of extra cash from month to month. She'd have to be on her own most of the time here in his home office and a receptionist wouldn't bring in anything but extra work for him. She'd pretty much drain his bank account. However, he'd placed the ad, so he'd better follow through.

He sighed again and stood up. After a long stretch, he felt better and moved out from behind the desk. He'd spent the whole day inside, when what he liked the best was being outside in weather like this. However, he couldn't complain, he had all his bills paid for the month, he had food in the fridge and in the pantry and the roof over his head was paid for. Somehow, he'd find the money somewhere to hire the receptionist. He'd had enough people tell him he needed a live voice to answer his calls and to do it more frequently that once a week. His business couldn't thrive too long otherwise.

He looked at the clock: five o'clock was that early enough to be 'this evening'? Would Sandra Bernard call soon? He went in the kitchen and pulled a package from the freezer. He'd forgotten to pull out something to thaw at noon, so now he must stick it in the microwave for a few minutes. His mouth watered as he hit the defrost button. Nothing like a thick pork chop from the grill. That wasn't something that happened on the trail.

Colleen bustled around the kitchen fixing dinner. Ed would be home soon. Sandy sat at her easel in the conservatory, putting the last touches on her latest work. Tomorrow she'd take it and five others to the library. They'd hang them in her niche. Her heart thudded, she could take them herself in her own van! Charlie was downstairs she could hear his saw and knew he was working some intricate design with his jigsaw. She wished he'd take some of his pieces and put them in her gallery, she knew he could quit his post office job to go full time with his hobby, he was that good. She knew he wouldn't. For some reason, he loved being a walking mail carrier.

Only a minute later, a car with a loud exhaust drove up on the driveway and Sandy wondered what Ed would say when he came in after seeing her van. Before he came through the door her mom called, "Come on, Charlie and Sandy, Ed's home and supper's ready."

Sandy cleaned her pallet, threw her brush into the paint thinner and wiped her hands on a rag, then wheeled toward the kitchen. She was barely at her place when Ed walked through the door. His grin was directed across the table and he exclaimed, "Sis, you got your van!"

She grinned back at him. "Yeah! Isn't it great?"

"Super! When can you take me for a ride?"

"You come home sooner tomorrow and I'll give you an exclusive."

"I'll be here! Count on it!"

After Charlie prayed, Sandy picked up her napkin and a tiny paper fluttered to the floor. She couldn't reach it, but Charlie saw it, so he picked it up. "Hey, what's this?" He turned it over and said, "Here's a name and phone number. Mama, did someone call for Sandy today?"

Colleen nodded and mumbled, "Yes, while Sandy went to get her van that man called."

Sandy snatched the paper Charlie held out. "Oh! I wonder if it's for that job I applied for down in Georgia."

"I think it is," Colleen whispered.

"Super!" Sandy exclaimed. "I'll call right after dinner."

Barely above a whisper, Colleen said, "He won't be there tomorrow."

Much to Colleen's consternation, Sandy went directly from her place at the table into her conservatory after they finished eating. Ed sat at the table talking with his dad while Colleen cleared the table and started the dishes. It was relatively quiet in the conservatory, so Sandy picked up the phone and dialed the long distance number. It rang twice before a man answered. Sandy almost lost her nerve, but then she straightened her spine, she could do this, even if her mom was opposed.

She swallowed and said, "Hello, I'm returning a call to Mr. Ramon DeLord, please. This is Sandy Bernard."

"Ms. Bernard, this is Ramon. Thanks for sending in your application. Are you still interested in taking the job of receptionist? I see that you made the application over a month ago. I've been away for some time and just today went through my mail. I'm sorry it took me so long to get back with you."

The man had a very pleasing voice on the phone. He sounded to be about her age, but she wouldn't let that worry her or distract her. "Oh, yes, Mr. DeLord, very much! When could I come for an interview?"

"Let me see." Sandy could hear shuffling papers. "I'll be out of town through the weekend and into next week. The first day I have free is next Wednesday. Could you come in then? I realize you'll have to come some distance and probably have to stay overnight and weeknights are always easier to find lodging in this area."

Sandy was fast losing her nerve. She hadn't thought about having to stay over night. "You give me directions and a time and I'll be there."

A few minutes later, they hung up and Sandy smiled, then she grew sober. She hadn't had to tell him she was in a wheelchair, maybe he'd take one look and treat her like the wretched man at the car dealer. She'd definitely do without that, people like that made her angry.

Her conservatory was the center room and had two doors leading from it. Sandy wheeled first to one, then the other and closed the doors. She felt like playing and when everyone was home, even though she didn't make many mistakes, she only wanted to be background for conversation. She wheeled her chair to the piano, put the little black pouch in place and let her fingers glide over the keys. She hadn't played a new piece in a while, so she opened her Chopin book to the next Sonata. Soon, she was lost in the notes that her fingers transformed into music.

The other three people of the household were used to hearing beautiful music come from Sandy's fingers. Even so, Charlie stopped speaking in mid-sentence just to hear the beautiful tones coming from two rooms away. Sandy had certainly overcome her handicap. To look at her she was joyous with a smile for everyone. Her love of life soon made people forget that she was in a wheelchair. Her piano pupils loved her they would be heart-broken if she left. She also had a wide following in the city with her paintings. They were always in demand, but her playing, that she did just for herself was exquisite; he wished she could travel far with it.

Colleen finished the dishes and sat down in her chair at the table. She had a bit of embroidery to work on beside her place. Ed stopped for a breath and Colleen said, "What's she ever going to do if she takes a job so far away?"

Charlie reached across the table and took her hand. Her other hand stilled as she looked at her husband. "Mama," Charlie said, "let's not worry about it. She wants to be independent, to live her life. She knows she can't do that here. She'll find her place and we must let her."

"But she's crippled!" she sobbed.

14

Knowing how much Sandy hated that word, Ed came out of his chair nearly into his mom's face, when he said, "She's not either! She's handicapped, Mom. She got a van today that she can drive. She can go anywhere now."

"But she'll leave us," Colleen whispered.

Smiling at his wife, trying to reassure her, Charlie said, "Yes, Mama, she just might. She's a brilliant woman. She has talents that she can use anywhere. We mustn't hold her back, we must wish her Godspeed."

Snatching her hand from under Charlie's, she snapped, "I'll never do that!"

Shaking his head, Charlie said, "You may not have a choice, my dear."

Being the eternal optimist, Sandy packed everything she could fit in her van. Of course, she couldn't take her piano, but if she got the job, she'd find a place to live and have it shipped. It was Saturday, Ed and Charlie were both on hand to help load her things in her van and even Marcy was home to be a buffer between a very antagonistic Colleen and a very adamant Sandy.

When Sandy had ordered the van, one of the features had been that the back seat folded down into a small bed. Since Sandy wasn't tall, her legs hadn't grown in the same proportions as the rest of her body from her waist up, she could sleep comfortably on that bench. She knew she must stop between Philadelphia and northern Georgia for the night and she was determined to enjoy some of the sights along the way. She'd lived a very sheltered life so far and she wanted to see everything possible between here and there. She had determined that if she drove highways instead of interstates she'd see a lot more.

By noon everything was loaded. She and Ed had put the bench down and made it into a bed so she wouldn't have to do that alone somewhere tonight. Marcy carried her cooler with the sandwiches and ice water and put it down behind the console between the front seats. Colleen still stood on the back porch, tears flowing down her cheeks. Charlie wasn't saying much, but he had a smile on his face, even though his eyes were exceptionally bright.

The lift was down, but Sandy went up the ramp one last time and reached up to hug her mom. "Mom, I love you. Don't ever forget that. I'm not going away because I don't. I do need to act like an adult and be on my own. That's why I'm going." Colleen surely knew what Sandy wasn't saying. It didn't take a rocket scientist to figure it out and the others in her family knew exactly why Sandy was leaving.

"Oh, Sandy," she said, between sniffles and hiccoughs, "I wish you didn't feel like you had to do that. We know you're an adult. We love you so much."

"I know." Sandy kissed her mom then rolled down the ramp to her dad. He bent over and she hugged him and said, "Daddy, take good care of Mom, she'll be alone most of the day, you know. She may clean the daylights out of the place."

Charlie's eyes glistened, but he chuckled and kissed her on the cheek. "I'll do it, Honey, she needs keeping in line, you know. You drive safely and give us a call when you arrive. We want to know everything as soon as it happens."

"I'll remember, Daddy." Sandy kissed him.

Taking a deep breath, she moved to her big, little brother. She put her hand on his arm, he didn't like kissing his sister. "Ed, study hard. I know it's only summer school, but you want that teaching job and it's stiff competition here in the city."

"Believe me, I know that! I have my summer cut out for me. You take care, Sis. We'll be thinking about you all the way."

"Thanks." Last but not least, Sandy smiled at her kid sister. Marcy was in nursing school downtown. She'd make a good nurse she was dedicated and had a vision. "Marcy, study hard, but don't let all those doctors distract you much."

Fiercely, Marcy answered, "I wish I was going with you!" Both sisters looked up the ramp at their mother. "Mom can be so...." she whispered.

"Yes, but come home and love her often, Marcy, she needs you."

"I'll try, Sis." *How could Sandy be so positive about her mom's treatment of her?*

Sandy was on the lift, but hadn't moved to push the button for it to go up, when Charlie said, "Shall we pray for you and your trip?"

"Oh, yes, Daddy, would you?"

Charlie looked up at Colleen, who still stood on the back porch. She had dropped her head and closed her eyes, so he turned to his three children and held out his hands to his two daughters. They each took his hands, then grabbed Ed's hands to complete the circle, bowed their heads and waited, the silence was only broken by Colleen's sniffles.

"Father in heaven, Sandy has an interview in a few days in Georgia. She has many miles to travel to be there. We pray that You will take her safely and give her a good interview with this man. If it is Your will that she get this job, we pray that she will do a good job for him. If it is not Your will for this job that You'll bring her back to us safely. Thank You for keeping her in all she does, we love You completely. We pray in Your Son's matchless name, Amen."

Fervently, all three in the circle said, "Amen!"

Charlie, Ed and Marcy stepped back as Sandy took the controls and raised the lift, then wheeled herself inside the van. She turned and raised the lift to the traveling position and closed the outside door. When it clicked shut, Sandy moved to behind the wheel, locked herself in place and pushed the key into the ignition. Butterflies were diving into the walls of her stomach as she turned the key and the engine purred to life. Colleen stayed on the back porch, as if staying there would keep her daughter from leaving. Sandy waved and as the other three waved back, she backed down the driveway. Colleen wouldn't watch and she wouldn't wave. Charlie, Ed and Marcy followed Sandy, then as she turned on the street, they waved until she made the turn on the Avenue through town. They looked back, Colleen still stood on the porch weeping.

Sandy sighed as she looked in the rearview mirror and saw three of her family waving. Why couldn't her mom be supportive? Yes, she was handicapped, but she wasn't an invalid, she'd never been one to be pampered. She turned from their relatively quiet residential street onto the Avenue through their part of the city and joined the traffic headed downtown. She didn't have much experience driving in city traffic, so she didn't like the city streets very much. It was quite a ways to the Schuylkill Expressway, but she was no wimp, she'd do just fine.

By the time Charlie, Ed and Marcy reached the back door Colleen was inside and had shut herself in the bathroom. Ed and Marcy looked at Charlie, who looked at the shut bathroom door. He looked back at his other children and shrugged. "I guess we'll wait for her to come out. Go do whatever you were going to do this Saturday."

"I got studying, so I'm off to my desk," Ed answered. He turned and headed through the mud room into the kitchen, on the way to his second floor room.

Marcy sighed, "This is my first day off in two weeks, I brought home everything I own and it's all dirty. I'll be most of the day doing laundry."

Charlie chuckled. "Have at it, girl, Mama did ours yesterday."

"Thanks, Dad, I will."

Ever since he'd talked with Ms Bernard, Ramon thought about her. She seemed excited to take the job. She didn't sound old, but her voice sounded mature. After he'd talked with her, he'd had two, three day trips scheduled. The one he was doing now was from Thursday through Saturday, the next was with two couples from Sunday through Tuesday. They'd get back in the evening before supper. He'd have time to get his clothes and gear cleaned up and ready for his next trip starting Thursday, with the interview on Wednesday.

If she took the job, he wondered when she could start. She probably had to give notice to the place where she worked now. In a few days it would be the first of August and the weather only let him do these trips through October. That was three months. Was that long enough to warrant a full time receptionist? He shrugged, maybe she wouldn't work out. She would have to find a place to live and his little town didn't anything in the line of housing or vacant apartments. People who were here, lived here a lifetime....of course, there was always Isabel's cabins.

It was late in the afternoon and they needed to pitch their camp for the night. They'd be back to home base tomorrow, but tonight was supper and a small campfire. He began looking for a good place to stop. One couple had a tent, but the other and himself slept out under the stars with a campfire to keep the mosquitoes away.

"Here!" one of the girls exclaimed, a few minutes later. "Isn't this the perfect place for a camp? Look at the view! You can see for miles."

"Yeah," her friend said, enthusiastically. "Can we set up camp here, Ramon?"

"Sure! I was starting to think about where to set up, but this is as good as any place. There's even a stream for water."

"Great!" one of the men said, "Alex and I can set up the tent while the girls go filter some water for our supper."

TWO

Sandy had never been a long distance from Philadelphia. Her aunts and uncles all lived on a dairy farm north of the city and supplied some of the milk for the stores. She visited them when her family did. Her dad always worked to support them and her mom had always stayed home, home-schooling her while her brother and sister attended public school. Now both of her siblings were in higher education on scholarships and her dad didn't need to work quite so hard, but he was from the old country and his work ethic was awesome. Sandy admired him and as much as her handicap allowed, she tried to emulate him and he had encouraged her.

When she had finally seen the last of her family, she paid close attention to the signs and finally left the city streets for the interstate that the locals knew as the Schuylkill Expressway that went downtown and linked with the interstate that took her away from Philadelphia. When she finally left the city and found more space, she breathed a sigh of relief, she had made it, her hours of studying the atlas had paid off she hadn't gotten lost in the city. Of course, there were still several hundred miles where she could get lost between here and her destination of northern Georgia. She planned to take her time, since today was Saturday and her interview was for Wednesday, she could sightsee along the way.

As soon as she left the city, she pulled out one of her sandwiches and ate it, then ate an apple and drank some water. She noticed her gas gauge needle was pointing to a spot that was dangerously near the 'E', so she found an exit with gas advertised and pulled off. This would be the first time she'd pumped her own gas, she'd filled up at the station close to home, but their friendly attendant had filled her tank for her. She tried to gauge where she should pull the van so she could reach both the pump nozzle and her gas tank, then stopped and shut off the engine.

Just as she opened the door to let down the lift, a car zoomed around the van to use the pump in front. Her heart jumped into her throat, she had her finger on the control to lower the lift when he flew by. Quickly, before another car came, she pushed the button and the lift started out from the van. Another car screeched to a stop when they saw her move out onto the lift. The car still bounced as Sandy lowered herself to the pavement. She intentionally didn't look at him, but the driver's mouth dropped open as she wheeled herself around the back of her van.

With her credit card in her left hand, she moved her chair as close as possible to the pump, but had to strain to reach where the card slid into the slot. Grumbling, she said, "I guess the inventers of these pumps never thought about a handicapped person wanting to pay for their own gas with a credit card." She followed the instructions and soon had her tank filling.

Just before the automatic shut off clicked, someone came around the back of her van and in a loud voice, said, "You need help?"

Sandy smiled at the man and said in a very normal voice, "No, I'm perfectly able to fill my own tank, but thanks anyway."

Uncomfortable, the man quickly turned away and said, "Yeah."

She turned back, when the nozzle clicked she pumped more gas into her tank as she'd seen both her dad and brother do. Since she ignored the man standing behind her van, he finally shrugged and left, deciding that she really could handle her own job. She finished pumping the gas, hung up the nozzle and reached for the receipt. Another car had pulled up nearly to her bumper, waiting to pump gas, so she went to the back of her van and looked, first at the tiny space, then at the driver sitting impatiently in his car with the engine running. He was too close to the pump for her to go to his window.

She pasted a smile on her face and said in a voice she knew wasn't the most Christian, "Mister, could you please back up so I can get around to my lift?"

He wasn't paying attention, but Sandy noticed that the passenger poked him he glanced at her, then at Sandy. She saw him swallow, pull his gear stick down and back up a few feet. Sandy smiled again then wheeled herself through the tiny space to her lift. Without looking at anyone, she propelled herself onto the lift then into the van. Finally, back in the driver's seat, she started the car and drove up to the building. She needed to use the restroom and she wanted something besides water to drink.

It was late evening when she found a pull off that the sign said was only a rest stop, there were no facilities. There were two huge trucks parked in the slots, the diesel engines were running, but she couldn't see anyone in the cab, the drivers were probably in their sleepers waiting for late night darkness before they went on their way. It was nearly dark after she ate the rest of her sandwiches and finished her water. She stretched out on her little bed for the night. Morning was soon enough to tackle Delaware and beyond.

Before she stretched out on the bed, another truck pulled up on her other side and she was glad that the doors locked on her van. She lay down pulled the cover she had conveniently close over her and rested her head on her favorite pillow. "Father in heaven," she murmured, "thank You for bringing me safely this far. I don't feel very confident right now, but I know You will be with me all along the way. Bless Daddy, help him deal with Mom. Help Mom to accept what I'm doing. It was hard to see her the way she was this morning there on the back porch. I've known she doesn't want me to go away, but You know she would keep me there beside her for all her life. Please rest her mind and give her joy. Bless Ed and Marcy, You know I love them. They're both studying so hard, give them clear minds, I pray.

"Father," she sighed, "bless this interview I have on Wednesday. May it go well, may he want me and may he accept me for who I am and give *me* a chance to do the job. I'm sure I can do the job and with You, nothing can fail. May he look beyond my chair and see me as the person I am. Thank You, Father, in Jesus name, amen."

It was dark in her van, the semi next to her had the small running lights lit around the cab, but that was all the light there was.

She closed her eyes and didn't wake up until the next morning when the air brakes on the semi next to her made their loud hissing sound. Quickly, she changed her clothes, slid back into her chair and took herself behind the wheel. The sun shone in through the windows, as she started the engine and left the parking area. She had to get to a restaurant soon there were some needs she couldn't take care of in her van. Only a few miles down the road was a brightly lit sign and right under it was a big restaurant. She pulled in and went straight to the restroom, splashed water on her face and brushed her teeth. Refreshed, she went to a table for her meal.

When she'd studied the map, she decided not to take interstates, even though they would get her to her destination quickly and efficiently. She wanted to see some of her beloved country along the way and by all means, she wanted to skip as many major cities as possible that, of course, included Washington. D.C. Perhaps on another trip she could stop there and see some of the sights, but this first time on her own, she felt better sticking to the less traveled routes. Going through Delaware was a good way to do that.

Attached to the southern end of Delaware was a peninsula that belonged to Virginia and at the end of that was the Chesapeake Bay Bridge and Tunnel. She knew the views from that bridge would be awesome. She was very glad the sun was out she didn't relish crossing that bridge when there was a storm. She joined the traffic on the road after breakfast and went south. This road was not an interstate and cars zoomed by her, but she didn't care. She had time to make her leisurely trip to northern Georgia and she intended to enjoy every mile, it was summer and the day was beautiful. She had a camera and stopped several times to take pictures she could later turn into paintings on her canvases. It would be very refreshing not to always have to paint the same scenes.

She slept in her van that night, it saved on her finances. She planned to get a motel room on Tuesday, so that she could be as fresh and clean as she could be and as rested as possible. She was so glad that the weather was good for her whole trip. She couldn't imagine pumping gas in some of those places in the rain.

She drove into Blairsville Tuesday afternoon. Ramon had told her that it was the largest city closest to his tiny town. She pulled off the highway and began looking for motels. There were several, so she chose one at random and pulled into a handicapped spot next to the office. There was a man behind the desk whom she could see through the window. She left the driver's space and wheeled herself to the lift controls. When the door opened and she pushed the button for the lift to move out, she saw the man jump from his seat and run around the desk to the door.

Before she could lower herself to the pavement, he came out waving his hands. He stopped in front of her van and yelled, "Hey, umm, we don't got no place for no cripple here."

Sandy hated that word. She cringed, but she tried to smile at the man. "Well," she said, in a normal voice, "could you direct me to one who does? I need a place to spend the night."

Waving his hand vaguely over his shoulder, he said, "Maybe some place like that. I seen a cripple over there onst."

"Thanks," Sandy said and moved back into her van. The man didn't watch, he stomped back through the door and slouched behind his desk. As the big door clicked shut, Sandy turned and saw him through the glass. She grumbled, "I hate people like that! I'm not mentally deranged, I'm not deaf or helpless, I just can't use my legs!"

She drove across the street and started the same procedure there. There was also a man behind the desk and she shuddered, wondering what his response would be when he saw the lift start to leave the inside of her van. She made it to the pavement before the man left his seat at the desk and came around to the door. Instead of barreling outside as the other fellow, he stood at the door and held it and smiled down at Sandy while she made her way up the small incline and went in the office. Of course, she smiled back at him.

"Hello, Ma'am," the man said, in a normal voice. "Are you needing a room for the night? Is there anyone with you or will a room with one bed be sufficient?"

"I'm alone, one bed is plenty, thanks." He nodded, accepted her credit card and wrote something in his book. "Oh, I almost forgot, could I book that for two nights?"

"Sure, Tuesday and Wednesday nights are no problem around here." He smiled at her. "The room I'll put you in is handicapped equipped. The shower area is large to accommodate a wheelchair, or there's a bench that pulls down to sit under the shower. Believe it or not, in the sink area is a small refrigerator and a microwave for your convenience. Our restaurant is also handicapped friendly and it's at the far end of the complex. I hope you enjoy your stay with us."

"Thank you, sir, you're very helpful. I appreciate your kindness." She nodded across the street. "Someone like you needs to give that fellow across the street some lessons in how to deal with handicapped people. He was very rude and almost obnoxious, if you know what I mean."

The man shook his head, looking out the window at the other establishment. "The owner of that facility lives in Atlanta. He runs a cheap ship, does as little for the facility as he can and hires cheap labor. I think they may have one room where someone with a wheelchair might be able to get around, but I'm sure it isn't much."

Sandy shook her head. "He came running out and yelled at me saying that he had no place for no cripple."

The man shook his head again. "I'm sorry he was your first encounter with Blairsville. Most of us aren't like that." He walked toward the door again. "Ms Bernard, your room is that one closest to the restaurant. Enjoy your stay."

"Thank you, I hope to, believe me." Sandy breathed a sigh of relief as she rode back onto her lift. A good bed would be a nice change from her bench.

It was late afternoon when Ramon and his hikers returned to base. One young woman threw her arms around him and exclaimed, "That was great! Thanks so much, Ramon! This trip was everything Al and I dreamed of. We'll call early next spring to book another hike."

Pleased, Ramon said, "Thanks, Jennie, I'm glad to know you enjoyed yourselves so much." He chuckled. "As of right now, I have a clean, white page starting next January. Of course, I don't book any trips until the very end of March, but you'll have your pick if you call soon after the new year."

"We'll do that," her husband said.

Ramon shook hands with the other couple and helped them put their gear in the back of their cars. He waved as first one then the other pulled out of his small parking lot onto the road back to Blairsville. They would have to travel at night to get home or book a motel room. He'd wanted to get back earlier, but where they'd camped last night had been too far away for that to happen. No one could travel fast carrying a huge backpack on his back.

He picked up his backpack and carried it over his shoulder to the door into his office. He kept a key for it hidden close by so he didn't have to carry keys with him. He didn't relish the possibility of loosing keys on the trail. As soon as he was in the office, he saw the light flashing on the answering machine. He wondered how many messages there were and how many were to book another hike. He only had a few slots left to fill before the season was over. He looked at the caller ID, none of them was from Philadelphia.

Without stopping to listen to any of them, he went on into his house, straight to his laundry room. All he did was unzip the large pocket and dump his clothes into the washer, add detergent and start the machine. Quickly, he stripped out of what he had on, threw them in the washer also then pulled out a robe from the basket of clean clothes still sitting next to the dryer.

He sighed, maybe his mom was right he needed to get a wife who'd do the cooking, cleaning and take care of the clothes. He guessed he really didn't have a life, at least not from April through October. Those seven months were about making money to keep his body and soul together for the other five months. His stomach growled and as he left the laundry room, a ray of slanted light told him it was time to shower, eat and go to bed. He'd start his supper, shower, eat and listen to the messages. The shower sounded especially good right now, so he hurried to the kitchen to see what was easy to fix.

Ramon took a large mouthful and chewed, then pressed the replay button on the answering machine. The first message was his mom, he made a face he hadn't called her the last two times he'd breezed through on his way to his next trip. He'd call after his interview with Ms. Bernard. The next four messages were prospects, so he took down names and phone numbers, he'd call them as soon as he finished listening to all of them.

The last message said, "Mr. DeLord, this is Sandy Bernard. I wanted you to know I'm in Blairsville and I'll be arriving at your office tomorrow at ten o'clock as we agreed. I'm looking forward to meeting with you."

"Yeah," he muttered, "I'm looking forward to meeting you, too. Maybe it'll work out and I won't have to do all this call back stuff myself."

He shook his head, he couldn't put off making these calls tomorrow, or saving them for her to make tomorrow, if she didn't work out, he'd be stuck with nothing and no time to do it then. He could call his mom tomorrow, he could do some chores around the place with the phone on his shoulder, but he couldn't book trips that way, he had to have his appointment book in front of him for that. He finished his dinner, took his plate and glass to the kitchen, rinsed off his plate, then refilled his glass and went back to his office.

When he went in his bedroom that night, he had his entire calendar booked solid until the end of October. As he lay down on the comfortable bed and pulled the sheet over him, he wondered at the wisdom of hiring a receptionist to run the office. The only thing she could say was, 'Sorry, he's booked full until he closes in October. Call back next year.' He sighed and closed his eyes and because the bed was so comfortable, he was asleep before the light on his bedside table was cold.

Sandy unlocked the door into the room she'd rented for the next two nights and wheeled herself in. Straight ahead was a sink just the right height for her. Below the counter she saw the refrigerator and on the far end from the sink was the microwave. If she stayed in Blairsville longer than two nights, this would be ideal. She couldn't, of course, the cost was prohibitive. The door to the right stood open and she could see the toilet with the arm rails on both sides. That would be helpful. As she pushed the door open wider, she saw what the man was talking about, the shower area had only a small lip that a chair could easily roll over, but that was high enough to keep water from the shower from flooding the room. It was spacious, easily accommodating a wheelchair. She wished her chair didn't have a motor on it, she'd love to sit in it and let the water run all over her. However, she saw the bench and knew she'd be using that tonight to shower and wash her hair. What a luxury!

When Sandy was a teenager, she'd complained bitterly that she couldn't get into the tub and take a real bath or a shower, so her dad and brother had rigged up a seat that she could swing over the side of the tub and maneuver herself onto. However, it wasn't the best arrangement and when she finished, she was usually exhausted. Most of the time she took a sponge bath at the sink, just so it wouldn't take as long or wear her out as much. Her hair was another matter. She was glad it had natural waves and didn't need to be washed as often as Marcy thought hers needed washing.

She made sure she had the key to the room in the pocket of her chair and wheeled herself back to her van. From the very back, she pulled her suitcase, set it beside her chair, closed and locked the door, then set the suitcase on her lap and went back inside the room. She smelled the aromas from the restaurant and that made her stomach growl, but she decided to shower first then make her way to the restaurant. Her stomach must wait, being clean and having on clean clothes was first priority.

After her shower, she noticed the phone on the bedside stand and saw that the area code and first three digits were the same as Ramon DeLord's number. She decided to call and let him know she was in town. Her fingers were shaking as she punched in the numbers. She straightened her spine, the man didn't know she was handicapped, why should he be reluctant to interview her? No one answered and she was relieved. When the mailbox opened, she was glad she could leave a message. He'd told her his only available time to give the interview was tomorrow, that he'd be on a hike today and again on Thursday. She hung up and smiled. Tomorrow could be the first day of the rest of her life. Or it could be just another day in her handicapped existence. No, she wouldn't think like that!

Finally, she followed her nose next door, pushed the glass door open and wheeled herself in. The hostess smiled at her and motioned her to a table where she had a wonderful view of a quiet park that was out of the main flow of people among the tables in the restaurant. It was a table for two, but the hostess immediately took one of the chairs away so that Sandy could wheel herself up to the table. She smiled at the woman.

Holding out a large folder, the woman said, "Ma'am, here's a menu, a server will be with you in a minute. I hope you enjoy your meal."

"Thanks, I'm sure I will." Sandy added to herself, *Whoever owns this complex has trained the help well. Everyone seems to know how to treat handicapped people. Everything about this complex is super.*

Wednesday morning, Sandy was up early. Just because it was so accessible, she took another shower then dressed in her best outfit. As a child, her mom had wanted her to wear dresses, but she'd always been so conscious of her legs and how small and spindly they were. Once she'd reached her teen years, she'd insisted on wearing slacks for dressing up or jeans for around the house. However, she had several dresses and skirts she wore to church or for special occasions. The skirt she put on covered her legs down to her ankles and with the top she always combined with it, she knew she looked good. Drawing a brush through her hair, she sighed, this was as good as it got.

After breakfast, she hurried to her van, pulled out her directions and read them through once more. She must take the road out front out of town to the east five miles and make the turn on the smaller highway that led to her destination. Ramon had said that she'd better not blink too long or she'd miss Vansville, it was that small. She smiled as she fastened her chair in place and inserted the key in the ignition. She was on her way to her first interview for a job!

"Mom isn't here she can't put a wet blanket on this. If one gets put on it, it's because the man doesn't want a handicapped woman doing the job."

Ramon heard the alarm. Somehow, it fit into his dream, but the buzzing continued and finally rattled his brain enough that he woke up. He opened his eyes, realized he was in his own bed, smacked the clock to shut it off and reluctantly pushed the sheet off his body. The sun poured in his window, it would be a nice day and he could get a lot done around the place....

Then he remembered the interview.

Ms. Bernard had driven from Philadelphia for this interview, he couldn't lean in the car window, smile and say, 'Go on home, Ms. Bernard, I won't need you until spring. I'll hold the position for you.' *Yeah, she'll come back in March, I'm sure! Get with the program, man!*

He shaved, dressed and fixed some breakfast, then went into his office to take care of some bills and paperwork. He was still at it when a pretty light blue van pulled onto his small parking lot. He looked at the clock, time had gotten away from him it was five minutes to ten. This was Ms Bernard coming for the interview.

"Wow! It's ten o'clock!" he muttered.

He sat rooted to his chair as he watched the big passenger door slide slowly back. He squinted through the sunbeams until he saw the dark metal mechanism leave its position and start its slow movement from vertical to horizontal, then it hit him. "She's in a wheelchair!" he exclaimed. "I would never have guessed."

Thoughts rushed through his mind. Did he want someone in his office who was handicapped? She could probably answer the phone well enough. Was a handicapped person someone who could portray the image he wanted? *What are you, a snotty SOB?* a little voice asked from his shoulder. She would answer the phone, for goodness sake, not put on a dance show! He bunched the papers together he'd been reading and put them beside his blotter.

By now, Sandy was on the lift, but Ramon couldn't take his eyes away. She had sandy brown curly hair that glistened in the sunshine. Her face was lovely and the outfit she wore was perfect for a summer day. She pushed the button on one of the lift handles that brought her to the pavement. She pushed the little control on her right armrest and started toward the door.

Ramon grunted she'd be long since at the door before he reached it if he didn't unglue his rear from his chair and make for the door. In fact, he heard her knock before he'd reached the front of his desk. "Coming!" he called and hurried the rest of the way.

Ramon opened the door. From two feet, the lady was more lovely than by her van. Ramon swallowed, as Sandy smiled and said, "Good morning, Sir, I'm Sandy Bernard, I'm here for that ten o'clock interview."

Feeling like a jerk, Ramon stepped back and held the door so she could guide her chair over the threshold into the office. Finally, after another swallow, he said, "I'm pleased to meet you, Ms. Bernard, I'm Ramon DeLord." For the first time, he smiled and added, "I guess I don't need to offer you a chair, how about a glass of iced tea?"

Sandy chuckled and bumped over the threshold. "Sure, I'll have the tea. In summer one can't get enough to drink."

Ramon fled to the kitchen, pulled out two tall glasses then pushed them under the ice maker in the door of his refrigerator for some ice. He took the pitcher from the refrigerator and realized he couldn't offer her a refill. He shrugged well,… he did have enough for one helping each, so he filled the glasses and hurried back to his office.

Sandy still sat where he'd left her, but she was looking around at the pictures he had on his walls. "These are photographs you've had blown up?" she asked.

"Yes, these are some of my best ones. I've seen these places lots of times, but during the winter when I'm not on the trails I like to remember some of them."

"Are any of those places where anyone can get to?"

He opened his mouth, then realized what she meant, *anyone* being the operative word, translated meant *wheelchair accessible.* After a moment's thought, he said, "Umm, let's see, these were taken from trails that I've hiked, but there are some beautiful scenes close to where roads go. In fact, lots of the trails cross roads and scenes similar to these can be seen close by. Those roads wouldn't be hard to access."

"That would be super!" she said, excitedly. She wheeled herself closer to another picture and looked at it for a minute.

Ramon set the glasses down on a small table, gestured for Sandy to pull her chair up beside it, then sat in a chair opposite her. "I guess we should get down to the interview, Ms. Bernard. I have three weeks work to cram into today, so let's get started."

"That's fine."

"Do you have references?"

The light nearly went out in her eyes and Ramon wished he hadn't asked, but she answered, "Mr. DeLord, I have no references.

31

I've been self-employed up to this time, so I have only my accomplishments to recommend me."

"What would those be?"

She looked embarrassed, but she asked, "Are you into music or art very much?"

Shaking his head, as he said, "Only to enjoy the scenery around where I hike and on the radio while I drive, which is very little in the summer."

She sighed, "I'm afraid what I have to recommend me wouldn't help much."

"Try me," he said, liking the young woman and totally forgetting her wheelchair, which, of course, was her intention.

She shrugged, as if it was something anyone would do, she said, "I have been playing piano for some time. Six years ago I started giving piano lessons. My very first pupil now plays on a regular basis with the Philadelphia Symphony."

He nodded then it struck him. "You…" his hand came up and gestured toward the chair. He looked from her eyes, down to it, then back up to her face again. "You *teach* piano?"

"Yes." She didn't elaborate, but went on to say, "Also, at the public library in downtown Philly, there's a room I call my gallery. They hang my paintings there, except when they've sold out and I haven't had time to get in with more."

"Oh, my! No wonder you're so interested in my photos and the scenes I've captured with my camera. You do your pictures in paints?"

"Yes, oils, pastels and charcoal."

The phone rang and Ramon made a face. "That thing will be the death of me." He cleared his throat. "Ms. Bernard, before your call last night I had four others on my voicemail. When I answered them, I had booked my last free opening until I shut down my operation the last of October." He shook his head. "I can't book anything more until next spring, last of March, first of April. I should have thought of that when I talked with you and saved you a trip."

The light had come back to Sandy's eyes as she spoke of her piano and pictures, but now Ramon saw the light die completely with his words. Sandy's head dropped and she looked at the floor.

"I see." Her head raised after several minutes and she looked at him again. "So you don't book anything for next year? You don't book any kind of winter parties or excursions?"

Ramon scowled. "Well,....well, I haven't up to now. On a few occasions over the years I've been asked if I'd do one day outings in the woods or by vehicle to one of the area lodges and on rare occasions I have done that."

"Would you be able or willing to do that kind of thing?"

He shrugged, his hands fidgeting with a pencil from the desk. He swallowed, realizing that Sandy had put a lot of hope on this interview. He cleared his throat and said, "I guess I could on a limited basis. After all, I'm by myself in this. I'm gone all spring, summer and fall. I have things to do around here in the winter."

Looking anywhere but at Ramon, Sandy swallowed and said, "Sure, of course, I understand. I've booked a room in Blairsville for tonight. I'll drive around a little and see if I can find some of those scenes you mentioned and then head back to Philly tomorrow. Thanks for your time, Mr. DeLord."

"Umm, yes," he said, reluctantly.

She pushed the control on the armrest of her chair and moved agilely toward the door. Ramon hated that tone she had in her voice, but what could he do? Hire her to do nothing from now till the end of October when he really closed down? She had reached the door and was about to push it open, when he said, "Wait!"

She turned her head and looked at him. "Yes?"

Now what did he say? "Umm, my phone keeps ringing. People don't know I'm booked full. You could at least answer and tell them there's no more room. Of course, there is an occasional cancellation that could be rebooked." He left his chair and came toward her.

She looked up at him, he was a nice looking young man, well built, of course, that was due to his hiking. He also had a Mediterranean heritage. She smiled at him, but kept her hand on the control, as she asked, "How many calls do you think there'll be in the next two and three quarter months? Enough to pay me to tell them that?"

He came and stood behind her, prepared to open the door for her, he supposed. "I couldn't pay too much, I guess, but my friends tell me I need to hire another guide and I guess I could take on a few late fall and winter trips." His mouth closed, he didn't know what else he could say about anything.

She shrugged. "I arrived in town early and drove around a bit. I noticed there's a string of cabins down the road. If something like that could be rented and I could bring my piano down, I could paint and give lessons to support myself along with your pay, I think I'd be comfortable. The scenery between here and Blairsville was extremely lovely. Perhaps I could ship some oils back to Philly."

He touched her shoulder and she looked up at him. "Come back to the desk. I think we could work something out."

He moved to his desk and she rolled back. He sat down and pulled out a phonebook, not exactly sure why. After a few minutes thought he asked, "If you came in from say nine to twelve each weekday to answer the phone and whatever came in on the voicemail and took care of mail, everything but the bills, of course. If I rented one of those cabins for you, would that be payment enough? Could you make it for the rest of your needs with your paintings and lessons?"

She shrugged. "I have a bit saved, but it wouldn't last long. I'd need a clientele who wanted piano lessons. My paintings sell in Philly, but I drive my van wherever I need to go."

Ramon sat looking at his calendar that was in place of a blotter on his desk for several minutes. "Give me the number of the motel there in Blairsville. I have to be gone starting at eight tomorrow, but let me think about this and I'll call you later today or this evening. Will that work for you?"

Sandy had picked up a calling card from the motel, so she laid it on his blotter. "I'm in room one-sixteen, Mr. DeLord. I'm sure the person in the office can ring me. Like I say, I think I'll drive around to see some of this beauty until evening, so call after supper sometime."

"I'll do that, Ms. Bernard. Thanks for coming in and giving me something to think about. I'll get back to you later."

"Thank you for your time, Mr. DeLord. I'll be waiting for your call."

Sandy hurried to the door and had it open and herself through it before Ramon could get around his desk and the few steps to hold it for her. She let the door go and without slowing down, headed for the lift she'd left on the pavement. Without stopping until she was on the lift, she pushed the button and the lift started up. Ramon stood inside the closed door and watched her. Of course, all he could see was the profusion of waves on her head and the back of the chair. As soon as she was in the van, the lift started to go up. Soon, the door slid shut and he couldn't see her any more.

Ramon sighed, "Did I blow that, or what?"

As soon as the van left his parking lot, he went back to his seat behind the desk and punched the button to replay his messages. He'd had three calls while she'd been here and he hadn't taken any of them. He listened to each one, jotting down notes as he did. While the last one played, he realized if he'd hired her on the spot, she could have done what he was doing and he could be doing something else, something he needed to do before heading out tomorrow.

He knew what cabins she had referred to and before answering any of the messages, he flipped open his phonebook and looked up the number. When the lady answered, Ramon said, "Isabel, this is Ramon DeLord. Do you rent your cabins for longer than a day at a time?"

"Yes, Sony. I have several people who come for a month at a time."

"So you have rates by the month? Do you rent for longer than that?"

"By the month, Sony, but if you want it for longer, you tell me before the month is up and it's available for another month without moving out. Why, I thought you had your own place."

"I do, Isabel, but I'm hiring a receptionist and she needs a place to live. I know your cabins have kitchen facilities, so one of those would be ideal." Not thinking about her handicap until that minute, he said, "Are any of them big enough for a wheelchair to move around in?" He'd been in some of her cabins, two of them especially were quite small.

"Oh, sure, my number one cabin is quite large. It's also my best renter."

"I'll come by later on and pay for a month, okay?"

35

"That's fine, Sony. You're sure she's only a receptionist?"

Scowling, he said quickly, "Well, yes, of course!"

The old voice held some laughter, as she said, "As you say, Sony. I'll see you later on."

Ramon hung up and scowled, pushing back from the desk, he put his hands behind his head and his stomach growled. "Shut up," he muttered. He had too much to think about just now to remember that it was lunch time.

"Am I sure she's only a receptionist? What's that supposed to mean?"

Oh, she had hair you'd love to thread your fingers into. Her lips are perfect, even without makeup. Her skin is flawless and her face.... well, a goddess couldn't be more beautiful. Above her waist she's more perfect than many women you've seen, who haven't been in a wheelchair and her personality is so captivating you forget she's in a wheelchair. Not to mention she's extremely talented.... Yeah, well, she couldn't go on the trails with me. *You didn't want her on the trails, you wanted her here as a receptionist, stupid.*

Disgusted, he dropped his hands from behind his head, slapped the desk then jumped up, as his stomach growled. "Get a grip, DeLord. Get a sandwich and call your mom," he grumbled, looked out to where the van had been. He sauntered into the kitchen, opened the refrigerator door and stuck his head in. He had two crusts, one slice of bologna and two of cheese. His mayo was gone and the mustard container squeezed air at him. He definitely needed to get to the store or he needed a keeper.

"And that will not be Mom!"

Sandy didn't look back at Ramon's house. She was sure he wouldn't call and if he did, he'd say he was glad he'd met her, thanks but no thanks. She'd gone down the three streets of the little hamlet of Vansville before and discovered a grocery store, a post office, a gas station hardware store combination and a church. On the edge of town were the cabins she'd mentioned, but she didn't expect to need one, so she drove on by.

The tea had gone quickly from her mouth through her stomach, she needed to get to her room and let it come out. Fortunately, it wasn't far to Blairsville, so she relieved herself and changed into lightweight slacks and a cooler top then went to the restaurant for a sandwich. The clock on the night stand showed that lunch time was at hand. On the table in her room had been some brochures and she'd put them all in the van. After lunch, she looked at two of them and decided to do some exploring. Her fingers itched to grab her paintbrush and get to work.

She took the road that went back to Vansville, because there was an overlook where she wanted to do a painting. She pulled into it, then went to the back of her van and pulled out her easel, a canvas, her paint case, her pallet and brushes. Only a few minutes later, she was making the broad first strokes for the background. Sometime later someone stopped, but she didn't look around, she wanted to catch that soaring eagle that hung effortlessly over the valley.

Ramon called his mom, but said he couldn't talk. He had many errands to do before eight in the morning. On the way back from Blairsville, he started by the pull off he'd gone by hundreds of times, but this time, he saw a light blue van with the big passenger door open. About ten feet away, there was an easel set up and a woman working at it. As he looked a little more closely, he realized she had a built-in chair to sit in - it was a wheelchair.

He whipped in the far entrance and parked on the back side of her van. He got out and went behind his truck and her van and moved behind her. She was intent on her painting she didn't even glance at him. He looked in front of her at the scene she was painting and realized there was an eagle moving on the wind currents. He looked at the canvas and though the scene was mostly roughed in, the eagle was magnificent. He shook his head. She hadn't been here when he went to town, but twenty minutes later she had a picture recognizable enough for him to know the scene. No wonder she couldn't keep her gallery full! He hadn't even seen a finished product and he wanted to buy this painting. Even the few strokes she'd made around the eagle were perfect and the sun sparkling on the scene shone through on her work.

The eagle moved away on two graceful flaps of his wings and Sandy moved to another color and another spot on the canvas.

Ramon cleared his throat and said, "You are a master!" He didn't say her name, thinking she didn't know who was behind her.

"Thanks, Mr. DeLord. I love to paint and I've done it for years."

He came up beside her. "When did you realize it was me behind you?"

"I saw you come around my van. Thanks for not interrupting me when I was concentrating on that eagle."

"I was absolutely fascinated! No wonder your gallery runs out all the time! This picture is fabulous!"

"Thanks." She continued to paint, but never looked at him.

"Umm, would it be okay if I didn't call you, but told you here that I want you to come be my receptionist? I called the lady who owns those cabins. She rents them by the month and she has one that she says is large enough for a person with a wheelchair to live there comfortably. I'd rent it for you and buy that painting to start you off. Would that work for you, Ms. Bernard?"

She laid her brush down then turned to look at him. "Mr. DeLord, if you'll call me Sandy, I think I can live with those terms." She smiled and her eyes twinkled. "Did you come looking for me?"

Ramon had enough grace to look embarrassed. "No, no! I had some errands in Blairsville. On my way back I recognized your van, so I stopped when I realized you were painting. Umm..." his voice dropped, as he said, "my name's Ramon. I'd just as soon you called me that, too. If we're working together I think last names are too much of a formality, since we're about the same age."

"Great!"

She picked up her paint pallet again and moved the brush in one of the paint globs. "So you'd like me to be there about nine o'clock in the morning?"

"You'll be staying in Blairsville tonight and it's farther from there to my place than the cabins, but I'm supposed to be taking a group out at eight. I'd like to give you some information and a key before I go, could you make it before eight?"

She chuckled and her eyes danced as she looked up at Ramon again. "Of course! I used to be the one who rousted my sister out of the sack for school when she was a kid. I'm used to early mornings I'll be there, say seven thirty, quarter of eight?"

"Yes, probably closer to seven thirty, that way we can have those things all done when the hikers need to suit up."

"I'll be there. So, what do you want in this picture?"

He raised his eyes from Sandy reluctantly, he realized he could look at her and enjoy himself for many hours, and looked at the scene beyond the parking lot, then said, "Oh, my! Just finish out that scene you're facing. I've often stopped here and looked out that way, but I've never seen an eagle in that spot."

"It'll have to dry, but I'll have it done today, Ramon."

THREE

Since Sandy wasn't looking at him, he said, "Thanks, Sandy, I'll see you in the morning."

"Sure, enough."

Ramon wanted to stay and watch her paint, but she put her brush to the canvas and began again, totally ignoring his presence. After several more strokes, he felt self-conscious and moved away. Sandy continued to paint, but she called, "Thanks for stopping by, Ramon and thanks for wanting to buy my painting. I'll see you in the morning."

He felt encouraged to move closer to her, so he said, "Sure, Sandy, I'm fascinated by your work and I'm anxious to see the finished product. I must get back home I have so much to do before the trip leaves in the morning." He sighed, "Not to mention those calls that came while you were there."

Putting another bold slash of color on the mountain, she asked, "Couldn't I take care of them in the morning? I'll probably have plenty of time for that after you leave. Surely I won't be answering the phone all the time. I'd rather earn my keep as sit around and watch the clock."

Ramon almost let out an audible sigh, he didn't really like those phone conversations. "Yes, that would be good. I'll leave them for you. Thanks."

Ramon went to his truck, started up and left the pull-off. Sandy continued to paint. She hoped Ramon didn't think she was rude, but the light changed so quickly she didn't want to lose what light she had. The scene was perfect with the sun shining as it was right then, but she could tell that soon the sun would be gone or nearly so and that would change the whole scene.

About an hour later, the light had changed dramatically, but she felt she'd finished the picture, so she packed her things, put them back in the van, except for the painting that she put on her lap when she wheeled herself on the lift. Before she closed the lift, she laid the picture on the back seat so that it would be safe from anything touching it and perhaps it could dry a little. Then she closed up the van and headed back to the motel in Blairsville. She took the painting into the room and put it close to the air coming from the climate control unit below her window. It would dry quite a bit before she left in the morning. She'd never had a painting bought before it was even finished, she hoped it was dry enough for Ramon when she went tomorrow.

She went for a shower, then dressed in another cool outfit and sat brushing out her hair there were some snarls from the wind at the turn-off. She looked back into the bedroom and saw the phone on the stand. She gasped, "I never called home! Mom will be frantic and Dad concerned that they haven't heard from me since I left."

Her stomach growled, but she decided to call first. She dialed out then put the call through and immediately her mom's voice said, "Hello, Bernard's."

"Hi, Mom thought I'd better call and tell you I got the job."

There was a long pause before Colleen spoke. "So you'll be coming home before you start?" she asked and Sandy could definitely hear the hopefulness in her voice.

Trying to hold in her exasperation, Sandy exclaimed, "Mom, of course not! It's a long ways to come home, besides, I start tomorrow. He's rented me a cabin close by as part of my pay, so as soon as my day is over for him tomorrow, I'll be moving in. I haven't seen the inside of the place yet, but I hope to send for my piano very soon. I don't want to get rusty, you know." *Haven't we been over this so many times already?* she wanted to say but didn't.

Colleen was choked up, as she said, "Sandy, why did you have to do this? Why couldn't you be closer to home, even commute to some place?"

Sandy swallowed they'd been over this so many times it was becoming like a broken record. "Mom, you wouldn't have let me take a job close enough to home that I could have commuted. You and I both know that. It's a wonder I had the chance to see that magazine long enough to get the application from it. Mom, you have monitored every piece of mail I've gotten since I was little except for letters that are sealed with a return address that you know. Mom, I'll probably come home for Christmas, but I'll have to let you know about anything else."

Colleen had tried to interrupt several times, but Sandy had continued to talk. When she finally stopped, Colleen immediately said, "I never....!"

"Yes, Mom, you did. Several times Dad's gotten the mail then asked if I'd opened the letter addressed to me, but I had to tell him I never saw it. I've seen you put magazines in the trash, then dump garbage on top before I could read them. Mom, don't deny it, it's true. Mr. DeLord's a nice man. I'm excited to work for him. I'll have time to do some painting and there are lots of places that I can paint. I'll probably keep my room at the library to show them."

Grasping at straws, Colleen asked, "You'll bring them home?"

"Mom, the pony express runs from Vansville to Philly every day. I've seen a FedEx and a UPS truck here since I came, so there are plenty of ways to get my paintings to the library in Philly. Anyway, as soon as I get settled I'll send you my address and when I get a phone, I'll send you that number, too. Take care of Dad and Ed, will you, but don't cook up too much, you know how Ed likes to eat."

"But how can you get your piano like you said?"

"I must see the cabin before I can decide, Mom. Staying in the cabin is the only option right now. The town is so small there aren't any apartments or places to rent other than the cabins. If it'll be too much in the way, I'll have to do without it, but I hope not. I'd like to find some students to teach."

"If the place is so small, how can you find students?"

"I don't know, Mom. It all hinges on getting my piano. Right now, I have this job and I can paint, so I'll concentrate on those two things." Sandy heard some noise in the background, so she said, "Is Dad there?"

"Yes, he's here," Colleen said, reluctantly.

"Oh, could I talk to him, please?"

It took a few seconds and Sandy wondered if her mom didn't want her talking to anyone else. Finally, Charlie took the phone and said, "Hi, Honey. So you made the trip okay?"

"Yes, and I got the job! I start tomorrow."

"It'll work out well for you?"

Her excitement projecting over the phone, she said, "Yes, I'm excited, Daddy! I get to work mornings in Ramon's office and then I have my afternoons free. I'll be moving into my cabin tomorrow, but I'm sure I'll soon be painting some of the beauty around here. In fact, I finished one this afternoon and the man I'm working for saw it and wants it. He'll pay me for it. It's drying by the air conditioner right now."

"That's great!"

Charlie dropped his voice and whispered over the phone. "Your mom was sure you'd be back as soon as you had the interview."

Instant tears came to her eyes, but she swallowed and said, "Oh, Dad…. It's the chair, isn't it? She was sure he'd take one look at me and turn me down."

"I'm afraid so, Sweetheart." He sighed, "I never thought she'd be like this."

"Daddy, I was sure she would be. Was there ever a time when she didn't think of me as a 'cripple'? I don't think so. When she couldn't keep me there in the first place, I knew she was sure I'd be home by now." *According to her mindset, no one would ever want me.*

His voice was normal again, as he said, "Well, my dear, do the man a good job and have fun. If you can paint some of the time, I know you'll enjoy your time there. I guess we'll look for you when we see you."

So glad her dad was so supportive, she nearly sighed. "Thanks, Dad. Say 'bye' to everybody for me and tell them I love them. Oh,

I hope to send for my piano, so you might look into movers if you can. I told Mom, but she probably won't even try."

"I will, Sandy, I'll see what I can find out for you. I love you, too, Sweetheart. You take care and have a good life."

Sandy replaced the receiver and sighed. She knew her mom would be that way, she'd never wanted her to be out of the house, she'd wanted to continue to carry her even when she got too big and nearly broke her mom's back. Almost since she had learned to operate her own chair she'd had to appeal to her dad to get to do anything outside the house. As for taking piano lessons and getting art supplies, it was like pulling teeth. Only in the last few years had she and her family and her aunts been able to convince her mom that she could function in the outside world. Colleen had fought each step Sandy had tried to take on her own. Was it any wonder she wanted to get far away? Before her agitation level rose any higher, Sandy turned on a light and left the room, then went next door to the restaurant for her dinner.

Knowing she must leave very early in the morning, she was glad she hadn't unloaded anything except her one suitcase into her motel room. She finished her supper and went back to her room. She laid out her outfit for the next day then packed up everything she wouldn't need in the morning. She would be ready to leave by seven. She would not be late!

Ramon went home and his answering machine was blinking. He almost reached for it, but decided to let it go at least for a while. He looked at the desk, but smiled when he saw the notes sitting in the middle of it. He didn't have to take care of them, Sandy would make them all go away even whatever was new on his machine. He shook his head he couldn't believe how exquisitely she had portrayed that eagle this afternoon. He had never seen a scene portrayed as exquisitely as she had done on that painting.

He looked around his office for a minute to find a good place to hang his new picture. It needed the most prominent place, because it would be by far the most beautiful of those hanging in his office. Besides, if he hung it where most everyone could see it, he might help Sandy sell more and that would help her. The phone rang, but he didn't answer, he let the answering machine pick up.

However, he stayed to listen to the message. The leader of the group that was coming in the morning, said, "Mr. DeLord, this is Tom Ramsey. We've run into a snag and we won't be able to get there to start at eight o'clock. Will it be…"

Ramon snatched up the receiver and said, "Yes, Mr. Ramsey, I just arrived back and you caught me. You won't be able to get here to start at eight?"

"Yes, that's right, Mr. DeLord. If we could make it ten o'clock or even eleven, we'd be in good shape. Would that be okay with you?"

"Sure, that's fine. I hadn't planned to leave town without you."

The man on the phone chuckled. "Yeah, I guess our presence is required, isn't it? We'll see you around ten or so, then."

"Thanks for calling, Mr. Ramsey."

"Sure, I'm glad it'll work for you."

Ramon looked at his watch and decided to eat then call Sandy. With two hours more time in the morning, he could meet her at her new cabin and help her move her things in. Even though he was sure she'd be able to do it herself, surely she wouldn't refuse his help. As he began his meal, he stepped back from the refrigerator and stared out the kitchen window. *DeLord, what's going on with you? You* want *to help Sandy move in?*

About an hour later, the phone rang in Sandy's room. She scowled, wondering who would be calling. She hadn't given her folks the number, only Ramon had it. What would he want? "Hello?" she said, tentatively.

A rich baritone voice said, "Sandy, my group for tomorrow called to say they can't be here before ten. If you came at the same time and stopped at the cabin office, I could meet you there and introduce you to the lady and give you a hand, if you'd like, before we had to get things squared away here."

"That sounds good! I'll meet you at the cabin office around seven thirty in the morning."

"Great!" *You don't know how much!* he said to himself.

Sandy hung up with a smile on her face, brushed her teeth and went to bed. She turned over on her side toward the window and looked at the painting that she had completed only a few hours before. It was beautiful, even if she did say so herself. She wondered where he'd hang it, in his office or his house. If he hung it in his office she wondered if it would help her to sell some around here. She shrugged and went to sleep.

Morning came along with clouds. Sandy looked through the crack in the curtains and made a face. It wasn't raining yet, but the clouds looked low and heavy enough to start any time. She hurried to dress, packed up her things quickly and put them in the van, then was the first one in the restaurant for her breakfast. She got herself in her van and it hadn't started raining yet. She could only hope that it would hold off until she got all her things in the cabin. Nothing she had would melt, but her canvasses wouldn't give as good paintings if they were wet.

She smiled, looked at the dash clock as she pulled out of the motel parking lot in Blairsville. She'd be early to her meeting with Ramon and he needed to know she was punctual. Actually, he had the same idea and they met as they turned into the parking lot for the cabin office. He grinned he'd gotten there a minute before her and pulled in ahead of her. He parked and left his truck while she pulled up beside him and shut off her engine. Just as she pulled the key from the ignition, he looked at her and shook his head. When he reached her door, she rolled down the window. She scowled, but he said, "Hi! That was perfect timing, wasn't it?"

"I'd say. However, I'd planned to be here first."

He laughed. "That was my intent, so I guess that's why we pulled in at the same time. It'd be easier if you drive to that first cabin, that'll be yours. This gravel isn't easy to drive your chair on is it? I'll bring Mrs. Isaacson over and introduce you. I called her after I called you and told her our plans."

"I'm with you on that!"

Before Ramon even finished speaking with Sandy, the older lady came out. As soon as Ramon saw her, he turned and waved to her. Sandy looked at the lady for several seconds, she had salt and pepper hair, with most of it in a bun at the back of her neck, but there were some soft waves around her face that made her look loveable. She wasn't fat, but a little plump, she reminded Sandy of her oldest aunt and her smile was captivating, making Sandy smile. Sandy looked beyond her to her house and noticed there were three steps but no ramp. Good or bad, Sandy could never visit in her home. Most people didn't have ramps up to their front door and to build one for one visitor was cost prohibitive.

When Ramon waved, the lady smiled. When Ramon left her van, Sandy put the stick back in drive and went the few yards to the parking space for the cabin where Ramon had directed her and parked so her lift came down onto the sidewalk. The sidewalk to her cabin went at right angles to the other sidewalk, giving her plenty of room to lower the lift and get herself off. Ramon hurried and was at the big door when Sandy put the stick in park, then he waited for her to get herself out. By this time, Isabel was on the walk, smiling at the young lady.

As soon as Sandy was on the walk, Isabel came over, waved her hand, as if to dismiss Ramon and said, "Hi, I know him, so we'll forget him for a bit. I'm Isabel Isaacson and I gather you'll be in this cabin for at least a month."

Sandy held out her hand. "I'm Sandy Bernard and I'm pleased to meet you, Mrs. Isaacson. Yes, that was my agreement with Ramon. I'm anxious to get settled in."

Isabel looked up at the leaden sky and said, "Come this way. This cabin is the easiest one to get to and is handicapped equipped, so I hope it's comfortable for you."

Sandy looked at the cabin it was definitely much bigger than the others. It had a large parking area with no curb from the parking place to the walkway to the cabin. She also noticed that it was much wider than any of the other walkways. Sandy followed the older lady up the ramp onto the large porch that ran across the entire front and Ramon followed her.

Isabel opened the door, then handed Sandy the key and said, "Here you are, Deary! My husband had this cabin built especially for someone like you."

Sandy smiled, took the key and wheeled herself inside. Ramon followed her. They looked around the room and saw that it was a nice sitting room. At the far end was an archway that showed a nice kitchen area and through another opening in the back wall was a bath. Off on the wall closest to the kitchen was another door that Sandy thought could possibly be a closet. There was still another door, but she couldn't see in the room.

As she looked around, Mrs. Isaacson said, "The bedroom has a full sized bed. I had the bathroom changed a few years ago so the shower is a walk-in, or drive in as the case may be."

As Sandy wheeled herself to the bath, she asked, "Is there a bench I can put down? You see, I can't take my chair into a shower, the motor there on the back can't get wet, but I truly enjoy a shower, Mrs. Isaacson."

The expression on the older lady's face showed how unhappy Sandy's question made her, "I never thought of something like that! I'll call my handyman today and ask him to put something like that in for you. Does there seem to be anything else?"

Sandy wheeled herself to the closed door and opened it, very happy to see that it was a closet and large enough to accommodate her chair, but the clothes poles were low enough that she could hang her things without having to strain. At the back was a dresser. There was plenty of room to store her paints and other supplies on the other side from the clothes out of sight.

From there, she went to the kitchen. It was much smaller than the one she was used to at home, but she'd known for a long time that her mom's kitchen didn't have to be what she gauged her own by, she could do with one quite a bit smaller, as long as it was big enough she could move around in it. This one had a refrigerator that was big enough, but not so big that she couldn't reach in the freezer and the stovetop was lower than a conventional stove.

She smiled at the older lady and said, "No, Mrs. Isaacson, this looks really good. If you don't mind, I have my own piano that I'd like to send for."

That was the first time the older lady looked from her to the wheelchair, then back, before she said, "You play piano?"

"Yes, I do, I have for many years and I also teach piano. If you know anyone who would like to take lessons, I'm pretty reasonable and I'd like to get back into the groove as soon as my piano can be shipped from Philadelphia."

"I'll keep that in mind." She still looked dubious, however.

Ramon wondered what else Sandy needed to make this place into her home. From the way she talked, everything she cared about was in her van except her piano. He glanced at his watch, time was slipping away, but he knew Sandy had to have things to her satisfaction or she couldn't be comfortable. He watched as Sandy sat looking around the room and wondered what else she needed to change. He knew she didn't need a full sized bed, but maybe she did.

Sandy moved to the bedroom and moved herself into the room. She hated to ask for something else, but she knew if she was going to live here indefinitely she had to ask, so as diplomatically as possible, she said, "Mrs. Isaacson, I'm sure the large bed is comfortable, but it's hard for me to get down so low and almost impossible to get back up. Could we maybe trade it for a daybed with pillows?"

"I have one of those in my attic," Ramon said, immediately. "I took it out of the room I use as my office. I'd have to move it right away, since my tour is coming at ten, but you're welcome to use it, since I have no use for it."

Sandy turned sparkling eyes on him and he nearly melted away. "That'd be great!"

"We'd have to move the bed out," Isabel said.

"Is there anyone around to help do that?" Ramon asked, knowing he could help, but these two ladies couldn't.

"I'll call my handyman right away."

"I'll empty my van while you do, then we can go to Ramon's and load up the daybed."

Ramon shrugged. "Sounds like a plan!"

Surprising both Sandy and Ramon, Isabel pulled a cell phone from her pocket and dialed a number. After the call, she came to the door to hold it open as Sandy and Ramon came in with armloads of things from Sandy's van. "He'll be right over. He also has a daybed that he said he can bring with him. We can trade the bed for the daybed in one move. That would be a better idea than to use yours, anyway, Ramon, since it looks like it'll rain any minute now."

Ramon looked at the clouds and said, "Yeah, you may be right."

Sandy and Ramon were bringing in the last things from Sandy's van when a pickup pulled in beside the van. Isabel moved furniture out of the path that the men would have to take to leave the room, while Sandy took her suitcase into the large closet. Ramon met the man at his truck and they took the parts of the daybed from the truck bed. They put the bed parts on the porch, then came in and went to the bedroom for the large mattress. Soon the full size bed was loaded on the truck and the daybed was set up in its place.

Isabel looked at the single, much higher daybed and asked, "Sandy, are you sure you'll be comfortable on that?"

"Yes, Mrs. Isaacson, that's what I've slept on at home for a very long time. It's been really hard to get out of bed the last two nights at the motel."

"Well, then, that's fine."

Sandy put the key on her ring and brought up the end of those leaving the cabin. Isabel went back to her office the handyman followed her, while Ramon went with Sandy back to her van. He stood on the parking lot while she lowered the lift and wheeled herself on it. They left the parking lot together and soon entered Ramon's parking area. The clouds were still ominous, but they hadn't opened up yet.

When they met on the lot again, Sandy said, "It's not a very nice day for you and your group to start a trip, is it?"

Ramon glanced at the heavy, dark clouds again. "No, but I tell each group when they sign up to be sure to bring some rain gear. We aren't the desert around here, we do have rain and this time of year we sometimes get rain from hurricanes that come up the coast. I listened to the extended forecast over breakfast and it's to clear tonight and be nice the rest of the week. We'll be back Sunday, so I'm sure it'll be fine."

Ramon held the door to his office for her and Sandy wheeled through. After it closed, he worked a key from his ring and held it out to her. "You're getting a lot of keys today, but here's a key to this door. I usually keep the door into the house closed, but not locked." He sighed, "That's only because I'm not a very good housekeeper." He shrugged, "But I live alone, it's not like I must keep up appearances." He nodded toward the far door and said, "Let me show you the bathroom. I'm sure there'll be times when you'll need to use it while you're here working."

She nodded. "I'm sure that's true."

She accepted the key then followed him to the back of the room. When he opened the door into the house, she knew immediately what he meant about not being a good housekeeper. The home she'd lived in was immaculate in comparison, but that was because both she and her mom were at home much of the time and could keep it picked up. Ramon was only home a day here or there. Keeping his house clean wasn't at the top of his priority list.

His house was all on one level and the room they left was at the end of a long hallway. There were two closed doors down the hall a little across from each other and Sandy assumed they were bedrooms. Just before the hallway ended was an open door and Ramon stepped passed it. Sandy looked in then wheeled herself into the room. It was barely big enough for Sandy to get her chair between the tub and the counter to the toilet, but she could, so that was all that mattered. The bathroom was set up differently from the one at her home, but it was about the same size. It would work just fine. Of course, she could not turn around in it.

He pointed on further to the kitchen, dining room and the living room, but Sandy knew she'd have no need to be in them, so she didn't go that far. They seemed fairly good sized, but her job was from nine until twelve each day, she could pack a lunch or go to her cabin if she wanted to eat there. She wouldn't eat his food. They had barely returned to the office when three cars pulled onto the lot and car doors slammed, but the rain still hadn't come.

Sandy looked out the window and said, "Looks like your mission is upon you, Ramon. I'm sure you're champing at the bit to get on the move."

Ramon sighed, "It's about this time of year that I wish I had someone else to send out, but maybe that'll happen next year. Let me show you quickly what's on my agenda."

She looked at him, her eyes dancing. "I think that's what we were supposed to do before these folks descended on us."

"Mmm, I think you may be right." He opened a book then set it down beside his blotter. Showing her both of them, he said, "I keep my bookings in two places in case one gets smudged or something,

I have another copy. Of course, the only way you'd be able to take another booking would be if one of these calls to cancel."

"Okay. Suppose someone calls while you're gone and wants to make a reservation for next year or after October, what do I say?"

"For next year, take information," he shrugged, "I guess do the same for both. I've not done it before, so it'll be new for both things. Make a tentative agreement and tell them we'll get back with them later, more into the fall, to firm up dates. At this point that's the best I can do."

She smiled, but saw the people approaching. "I'll do my best to keep it straight, Ramon."

Ramon was still bent over Sandy's shoulder and really wanted to kiss her. *Where had that idea come from?* However, the first people burst in through the door, so he straightened immediately, but kept his hand on her shoulder. When they saw Sandy at the desk, with Ramon so close, all three of the people came to a sudden stop and stared at them.

Ramon smiled and said, "Hi, folks, glad you're here." *Probably more than anyone'll ever know.* "Actually, I'm explaining things to my new receptionist. It looks like you're eager to get underway. Folks," he said, as the others appeared in the doorway, "this is my new receptionist, Sandy Bernard."

Sandy smiled and said, "I hope you folks don't mind getting wet. It sure looks like rain."

"Yeah, it does," the obvious leader of the group said, "but we all brought rain slickers, so we should survive and not melt."

Sandy laughed. "That's good! I hope you all have a good time."

Ramon said, "I'll be with you in a second. Everybody get your backpacks on and I'll be right out." They all walked out and he said to Sandy, "Should I call you sometime on Sunday when we get back?"

She looked up at him surprised. "Why? I think I can handle things. My cabin is perfect, I have a key to your office and I know what to say to anyone who calls and where to record everything. I think I'll be fine. Go and have a great time. This time you won't even have to think about the phone ringing off the hook."

He couldn't resist, he patted her back, wanting to do more, and said, "That's a relief, believe me. Remember, you don't need to be here Saturday and Sunday, even if I'm not back."

"I'll remember. Is that church on the corner any good?"

He'd turned away, but his head snapped back at her question. He scowled and said, "I have no idea, Sandy. I haven't been to church in years, probably since I was a tiny kid and it wasn't that church we went to when we went. Quite a few people from town go there, but that's not much help, I know."

Sandy smiled and said, "No problem, I'll make it. You go lead your group and try to dodge the raindrops when they come."

Ramon chuckled. "I'll try."

Ramon and his gang were hardly out of the parking lot when another car pulled in. This one blocked Sandy's van, she couldn't have lowered her lift if she had wanted to leave right then. A woman stepped out and came purposefully toward the door. Sandy, of course, didn't know her, the only woman she'd seen other than the women in Ramon's group was Isabel at the cabins. She watched as the woman came toward the door. She was totally different from Isabel, this woman was dressed to the nines, her hair looked like she'd come from the hairdresser and if she meant for it to stay that way, she surely had to sit up at night. Her nail polish matched her bright red lipstick and she wore spike, four inch stiletto heels.

The woman didn't knock she turned the knob and walked in. Sandy smiled and said, "Hi, can I help you?"

The woman stopped, scowled and asked, "Who are you? Why isn't Ramon there?"

"I'll answer your questions, but I asked you first. I'm Ramon's new receptionist, Sandy Bernard, and Ramon left with the group he was slated to take on a hike. Could I help you?"

The woman looked Sandy over, but because the desk hid her chair, the woman didn't notice Sandy was sitting in a wheelchair. "I'm Ramon's mother. I didn't think he had a trip again so soon. You say he left already?"

"Yes, a few minutes ago. I'm happy to meet you, Mrs. DeLord."

Disdain dripping from her voice, she said, "My name's not DeLord. That scoundrel of a man left me with a baby and a house full of debts." She waved her hands in true Italian fashion adding, "I'm Millie Casbah. He hired *you* to keep his office in shape while he's gone? Right?"

"I guess you could say that. Could I help you with something?"

She glared at Sandy, then at the desk, before she said, "No, but he must call me when he's back. He only called yesterday to say he couldn't talk. He said he had an interview and lots of errands. Since he had to leave today, I guess that makes sense."

"I'll have him call, Mrs. Casbah. I'm happy to meet you."

"Sure, I'll probably see you again. You're Sandy, did you say?"

"Yes, that's right."

The woman turned and left. Just as she closed the door behind her, there was a loud clap of thunder and before she reached her car, the rain was coming in sheets across the parking lot. Sandy was surprised that the woman didn't turn back and come in the office because of her hair and clothes. Instead, she raced for her car as fast as she could in her tight skirt and high heeled shoes and fell in. She slammed the door, but didn't start up right away. When the rain didn't let up for quite some time, she finally started her car, but nearly left tire tracks on the slippery pavement, heading down the street out of town.

Sandy shook her head. "I'd have never guessed Ramon's mom would look like that. She looks like a movie star and he... well, he looks like a hiking guide." Sandy didn't know Ramon's age, but surely he didn't have to report to his mom! However, she acted like he did.

The coffee Sandy had had for breakfast wanted to make an exit, so she wheeled herself into the house to the bathroom. Since the phone was quiet, when she was back in her chair, instead of going back to the office, she went on into the kitchen, inquisitive as most women are about a house. The sink had been in her line of vision when she left the bathroom and it overflowed with dirty dishes, she knew would smell awful before Ramon arrived back on Sunday. She rinsed everything and put things in the dishwasher, then started it. Of course, now that the sink was empty, it needed washing out and the counters needed wiping, so she took care of them, then wiped the table and straightened the chairs.

This room was on the back of the house. As she cleaned off the table, she looked out the window onto what used to be a garden, but was so over-run with weeds, nothing could grow. Sandy wondered if he'd grown vegetables or flowers at one time. Right now, nothing would survive with the weeds that were six feet high. She couldn't do anything about that, of course.

Sandy finished cleaning up the kitchen, but then remembered she had about six phone calls and messages to answer, so she hurried back to the office. She'd settled behind the desk when the phone rang. In as professional voice as she could muster, she said, "Hello, this is DeLord's Hiking and Camping Services. How could I help you?"

Sandy's voice was not squeaky or high pitched, but she was sure she didn't sound like a man she had never been accused of that. However, the voice on the other end said, "Ramon? Are you busy Friday or Saturday nights?"

Sandy said, "I'm sorry, but this isn't Ramon. He's gone with a group of hikers until Sunday. I guess that answers your question, doesn't it?"

After a pause, the voice said, "Who are you?"

"I'm the new receptionist, Sandy Bernard."

"Oh, well, just tell him, Stew called. Have him call me when he gets a chance."

"Sure, I'll do that. You have a good day."

"Thanks. Talk to you again."

Sandy hung up and sighed. She'd had two encounters since Ramon had left, neither of them very satisfactory. She picked up the notes that Ramon had left on the desk and sorted them. Obviously he wanted her to call and cancel or ask them to call back next year. She did as she was expected, but she gave each one the option to book something after the season closed. However, no one did. Perhaps they knew Ramon better than she did.

When she'd finished with the notes, she still had some time, so she went back into the house, deciding to straighten up the living room before she left. From the kitchen archway into the living room, she could see crumbs on the floor and the table beside a worn recliner. That was probably where Ramon ate his meals instead of in the kitchen, but as warm as the weather was and with his air conditioning turned off, those crumbs were a good calling card for bugs.

By noon, she'd cleaned up his living area and called all the contacts Ramon had left for her, plus answered two more that called while she was there. Several thanked her and hung up without making a reservation, one wanted to book a short trip in November and one wanted to schedule a trip in late March. She took the information and said they'd get back with them. She was anxious to get to her cabin and put her things away, but she wouldn't leave before noon.

She switched the phone to the voicemail and went to the door. She opened it and pressed the lock, but another clap of thunder brought a renewed burst of rain. She knew she'd be soaked by the time she opened the door, let down the lift, got on, raised the lift and wheeled herself inside the van. She sighed and waited. Ten minutes later the rain let up a little, however, she was tired of waiting, so she sent her chair into the fastest travel mode and headed for the van with her key ready for the lock. By the time she was inside, she was soaked to the skin. Even worse, she still had to get from the van to the cabin and make sure the van was locked.

She drove to the cabins and parked beside hers making sure when the big door opened the lift went down on the concrete of the walk. It was still raining hard, but she shrugged, she was soaked, what was a bit more rain going to hurt? She opened the door, put down the lift and wheeled on, then lowered herself. Quickly, she went to the back, inserted her key and sent the lift back up and inside, then put the other key into the other lock and closed the door. Rain dripped from her nose and there was a puddle in her lap as she turned to go up her walk. She shivered as a cool breeze swept through.

She pushed the knob on her chair forward as far as it would go, then was really glad there was a porch that could shield her while she got her key. However, instead of the regular door on the other side of the storm door being closed, she could look through the long glass storm door and there was a light on inside. She scowled, then tried the storm door and found it unlocked, so she went in. There was noise coming from her bathroom, she smiled, sure Isabel had asked the man to install the fold-out bench she'd asked for. Sure enough, when she wheeled over she found the handyman hard at work installing the fold-out bench. She smiled at the man's back, even though he wasn't aware of her.

"Hi," she said, "I'm sure glad you're doing that! I've had access to a shower the last two days at the motel where I stayed. I'm glad I can continue here, thanks to you."

The man nodded. "Isabel said she wanted this in today. I'm glad I could help make your day. It looks like you're soaked to the skin. Want me to leave?"

"No, I can go in my closet and change." She grinned at the man. "I wouldn't want you to leave and then forget what you were doing."

"I wouldn't do that, but I'll keep on and get this finished if it's okay with you."

"Sure, that's fine."

Before the man turned away, he pointed to the picture drying by the window and asked, "Say, Ma'am, who's the artist who painted that scene from the overlook? That's awesome!"

"I did. Ramon's going to hang it in his office when it's dry."

"My, my! When I first came in I thought it was a photo it looked so real. Isabel says you work for him." He shook his head. "You shouldn't be stuck in some office, you're a painter!"

"Thanks. I have been, but I felt I wanted to do more with my time. I'm sending for my piano. When it comes I'll give piano lessons. Do you know anyone who might be interested?"

The man looked Sandy up and down, including the metal chair she sat in. He had to know she was in it permanently, why had he had to install the seat in the shower and change the full bed for a daybed? Instead of answering, he said, "Say, I never told you my name and I guess you never told me yours. I'm Ted Lankaster and you?"

"I'm Sandy Bernard, from Philadelphia, but I'm hoping to make this my home, for now."

"You teach piano?" When she nodded, he said, "Put a sign in the window at the two stores. That'd get lots of attention. I really don't know anybody who'd want to play piano."

Sandy felt a chill go down her back, so she said. "Okay, I'll do that. I'd better get out of these clothes, so if you'll excuse me…."

"Sure, I'm almost done here."

Sandy was glad she'd put her suitcase in the closet. Now she wheeled herself in, turned on the light and closed the door. She took off her wet clothes and hung them over the rack, but the chair also was wet. She wished for another chair even if she had to stay in the closet, at least she could sit on something that was dry. She had nothing, so she blotted the canvas as best she could, then wheeled herself out of the room, just as Ted turned off the light in the bathroom.

Ted looked just a bit uncomfortable when he saw her, but looking in her face, he said, "Got her done. Why don't you go take a look? See if it's okay."

Sandy smiled at him and wheeled herself toward the bathroom. "Thanks, I'll do that." She wheeled herself to the small curb that kept the water in for the shower then went over it. Ted followed her and stood at the door. Sandy lowered the bench, then looked up to where the shower nozzle was and said, "This is perfect! It'll come right where it's supposed to. Thanks, so much." She looked a little bit further and said, "This is okay! Even the soap's handy. Thanks."

"You're welcome, Ma'am, glad I could do something for you. You know, those of us who have the use of our legs sometimes don't understand."

"You did great! And thanks for the daybed, too. I'd never get onto a low bed and back off. I need something much higher and more firm than that."

"I guess that's true. I'd never have thought about that." He shrugged. "So the bed is low, we just haul ourselves out of it, but we have strong legs."

"That's the size of it, Ted."

Almost as an after thought, Sandy said, "Say, Ramon couldn't help me, maybe you can. Is the church down the block any count?"

Ted shrugged. "Ms. Sandy, it's a church. That's about all I can tell you. I know for a fact hardly any men go there, but lots of the women go. My mom went there, but she found a better one in Blairsville, so that's where she goes. Me, I haven't gone in years. I take it literal it's my day of rest. I sleep in and eat brunch, then relax with the Sunday paper in the afternoon."

"Yes, Sunday's a day of rest, but God gave it to us. I feel we should honor Him by spending special time with Him that day." She smiled again. "Thanks, Ted, for fixing the seat in the shower so quickly. I really appreciate it. I also appreciate the use of your daybed, too."

"You're welcome, Ms. Sandy. I hope your stay here in Vansville is good. I can tell you'll be an asset to this place."

"Thanks Ted. I'm sure my stay'll be good." She looked out the window. "It's still raining. I was hoping to get to the grocery store today, but you saw how wet I got coming from Ramon's so I doubt I'll get there if it keeps up like this." She hadn't looked at the weather on the TV, was this some part of a hurricane?

Also looking out the door at the rain, Ted said, "Call 'im, he can deliver. My neighbor's a lady in her nineties and he delivers her groceries every week. Don't see why he'd refuse you."

Sandy nodded, as Ted opened the cabin door. "I may do that. It sounds like it's much less complicated than trying to go there myself in this rain."

Ted grinned and lifted his tool box a little. "See you!"

"Okay, Ted!"

FOUR

He slammed the door and Sandy was left alone in her little cabin, but she couldn't hear the rain, only see it. She was glad to be inside, but there were about nine people who were stuck outside not too far away. Would some of them chicken out and want to come back and then expect Ramon to give them a refund? She guessed she'd find out tomorrow at nine o'clock.

Sandy looked out at the rain. Since she'd left Ramon's it hadn't let up, but was pouring so hard she could hardly see the office. What Ted said made sense, but how could she call, she didn't have phone service she hadn't paid for one to be hooked up yet. She went in the kitchen and there was an old wall model hanging on the wall close to the sink. She shrugged no harm in trying to use it, so she lifted the receiver, shocked to hear a dial tone hum at her.

She dialed an 0 and was surprised when Mrs. Isaacson said, "Hello?"

"Hi, Mrs. Isaacson! I didn't know who I'd hear when I dialed I was shocked to hear a dial tone when I picked up the phone."

"Missy, if you want to dial out, you hit nine first then you'll get another dial tone. Since you'll live there, tomorrow you could call the phone company and they'll hook up a direct line for you. Did you want me for something?" she asked. "Did Ted get that bench to your liking?"

"Yes, it's great! I did want to get an outside line, so I'll do that now. I see a phone book here, so I'll use it. Thanks so much, Mrs. Isaacson."

As if she hardly knew how to respond to 'Mrs.' Isabel said, "By the way, since you'll be living here, why don't you call me Isabel?"

Smiling, Sandy said, "I'd love to, thanks, Isabel."

"No problem, Deary."

They hung up and Sandy started through the phone book. There were several towns in the small book and of course, Vansville was last. It didn't take many pages of the book to go from A to Z. She remembered seeing the grocery store, but she couldn't remember the name over the door. The book wasn't like the one back home businesses were listed right along with the private residents. Finally, she found it and jotted the number under the title on the back page for frequently used numbers. She looked back outside and the rain was still pouring down. She picked up the receiver again, dialed the nine, then the store number and waited. She wouldn't lose anything, all they could say was 'no'.

After the third ring, a man said, "Afternoon, Barkes Grocery, can I help you?"

"Mr. Barkes, this is Sandy Bernard. I've moved to town and rented one of Mrs. Isaacson's cabins. I was wondering if I gave you a list if there would be time this afternoon that someone from your store could bring it by. I'd pay them on delivery if you sent a bill along."

The gruff voice said, "Let's get a few things straight first, lady. I'm not Mr. Barkes, he died awhile back, I kept the name when I took over."

"I'm sorry, Sir, if I've offended you, I meant no harm," Sandy said, contritely. She took a breath, but the man seemed bent on vindicating himself and made a harsh noise.

As if she hadn't spoken, the man continued, "I got a couple old ladies who get their groceries delivered, but I can tell you aren't no old lady. This town's small enough, there ain't no reason an able-bodied woman of your age can't come and get her own groceries. Good day!"

Before Sandy could open her mouth, there was a dial tone in her ear. She took the receiver away from her face and stared at it. A tear slid down her cheek before she could check it. The man hadn't said 'no', but it sounded a lot more harsh than that. She couldn't imagine that calling him the wrong name had offended him, but obviously something about her call had. Slowly, she hung up and stared out the window. It had been several days since she'd eaten the last of the food she'd brought from home and the last two days she'd eaten at the restaurant connected to the motel in Blairsville, that's where she'd eaten breakfast this morning. From what she could remember in her quick trip around the town, there wasn't a restaurant in Vansville and her chair was still damp from her trip back from Ramon's.

She sighed, slowly replaced the handset on the wall and muttered, "I guess I can survive for three meals. It's good I ate a big breakfast back at the motel this morning." Sandy looked at the bare counter and saw the door to the tiny pantry standing open. The shelves in there were empty too. She didn't have to open the refrigerator to know that was also empty. She sighed she needed to get rid of her bad attitude. Maybe people did take advantage of a grocer during bad weather, but of course that hadn't been her intent.

She bowed her head and closed her eyes. "Father, forgive me for thinking bad thoughts against that man at the grocery store. When I think of the literature Marcy has gotten from those third world countries and how emaciated those sad children are, I know I will have no problem surviving for three mealtimes. Please bless that man, whoever he is. Also, Mom and Dad need Your touch, bless Ed and Marcy. Let them know I love them. In Jesus name, Amen."

Ramon led his group away. Each one had on a rain slicker, so they were a colorful bunch. The sky looked like it was bulging, ready to break open and dump tubfuls of rain on them. However, the group was in high spirits, so he decided they'd all survive, even if it did rain hard like it seemed it would. Not long after they left Vansville behind, they were in the hills on a trail heading out into the unknown to all except Ramon, who had traveled this trail many times.

From a distance they heard a grumble of thunder and one man looked toward the west, then at the black overhanging clouds and said, "It'll be raining here real soon. Look at the sky."

Ramon turned his head and said, "I'm sure it will. That sky looks like it's about ready to burst open at any minute."

The youngest woman said, "I guess my hair's destined for the wet rat department. Mom warned me that camping and hiking don't mix with salon styled hair. Like I'd know about that."

Ramon chuckled. "Your mom's pretty smart. I had a lady once who came for a hike, fortunately for her, it didn't rain, but she never went in water above her shoulders and she slept, or maybe she only dozed each night with her back against a tree and her hair in one of those bags like they have in the hospital. She must have had it done at the salon on her way to my office."

"Wow!" the young woman exclaimed. "She had to be exhausted by the end of her hike. I can't imagine her getting much rest up against a tree."

"By the last day, makeup couldn't hide the dark circles under her eyes."

"Makeup?" the girl giggled. "On a hike? She must have had a pull-behind suitcase."

"You should have seen the backpack her husband had to carry! I think she'd packed all her clothes along with his in his backpack and she had her cosmetics in hers. She even had a mirror. I do recall, though the last night she finally relented and slept in her sleeping bag and joined her husband in their two man tent. She didn't have her hair cover on, either."

"She had to be exhausted, doing all these trails in these hills. A mirror in her backpack?"

"Yes, she relied on all of us to get her safely over everything."

"What a dunce!"

Ramon heard another growl of thunder, much closer than the last. Up ahead about a half mile was a rock shelter, it would hold the women in the group and a rock overhang would shield the rest of them from the heavy rain. He quickened his pace, hoping the others would follow. However, the storm came faster than he anticipated and they were still a ways away.

"Uh-oh, it's upon us!" the group leader said. "I hear it coming up the side of this hill."

"I'm afraid so," Ramon answered. "Up ahead about a quarter mile is a rock overhang I was hoping to get to for some shelter. It'll give us some cover, but I'm afraid we'll be soaked before we get there. By the sound of what's coming we'll get a downpour." He glanced back at the four women and said, "You ladies will have your wet rat disguise in no time at all."

"Let's hurry!" the young woman exclaimed. "Wet hair isn't my favorite."

"Yeah, I'm sure you'll either have straight hair or curly."

One of the older women sighed, "Oh, to have naturally curly hair. I'd stand out in the rain all the time if I had that."

Her husband said, "You mean it's time for another perm?"

"It all comes out of a bottle, even the color."

Ginger snickered. "Maybe rain is truth serum." Ramon smiled, but made no comment.

The hikers followed closely behind Ramon. Even so, he couldn't see the rock formation when the rain overtook them. Before it hit them, a stroke of lightening snapped through the sky followed immediately by a boom of thunder. It was so deafening that some of the women clapped their hands over their ears. The noise hadn't even stopped when the rain burst over them. The women were hurriedly trying to cover their heads with some kind of plastic, but most of them didn't make it in time. Ramon didn't bother to say anything, he kept on hoping to see the overhanging rocks before the trail got so slippery they couldn't walk on it.

When they finally reached the rocks, the women rushed to the back and the men crowded in right behind them. Ramon stayed toward the front, he'd been on many trails when it rained, it wasn't something he liked, but he wasn't afraid even in a thunderstorm. Now that they were stopped, he thought for the first time about his new assistant. Would she stay her time at his office or with the rain would she rush back to her cabin? Knowing how slow the process would be for her to get from his place to hers, he couldn't blame her for leaving when she heard the first clap of thunder.

Behind him, he heard, "What if this keeps up all day? What do we do?"

Ramon turned and said, "It's up to you folks. We can rest a bit and hope the rain slacks up then move on or we can move on regardless. The other option is to go back and return your money and you'd still get wet. As you've noticed I'm sure, there are no covered bridges to help in that regard. Unfortunately, I have no time left in my schedule to reschedule this year. However, it's up to you."

"You're willing to take us on?" the group leader asked.

Ramon smiled at the older man as he wiped rain drops from his face. "Yes, I have no problem either way. As you can see, I haven't melted even though it's rained several times this summer when I've been on a trail with a group. From the weather forecast this morning, it's to clear off tonight and be nice the rest of the time we're to be out."

"We just won't make it as far now that it's raining," the man stated.

"Right. I'd planned to get quite a ways down the trail before making camp this evening. Even though we hurried to these rocks, we'll have to make camp closer than I had planned because it'll be slower going. It's no problem, though there are plenty of beautiful places and many good camping spots along the way."

The man looked around his group. "What do you say, folks? We either all go on, or we all go back. It's not an option to split up."

Looking around the group, as Ramon looked around silently, the man saw smiles, even from the women. Most of them nodded and even when another loud crack of thunder rang out over their heads, no one acted discouraged. He finally turned back to Ramon and said, "I guess we go on. Seems the girls don't even care if they look like drowned rats."

Ramon smiled back at him. "I guarantee if we go on their hair will be either straight or very curly." He chuckled. "To go back it would be, too."

Tom chuckled, "That's the truth. At least I'm not like some in the group, I have hair that can curl. One among us doesn't even have that."

The oldest man among them grumbled, "All right, I heard that."

By the time they stopped to make camp and eat supper, it was only drizzling and when they finished their campfire, the rain had stopped, but fog obscured any views. The group had brought several two man tents, enough for everyone in the group to sleep in a dry place. As Ramon spread his sleeping bag under a tree he wondered why he'd forgotten to tie his own tent under his backpack. The trees were still dripping and as he crawled into his bag, a large drip splattered on his forehead.

"Rats!" he grumbled. Probably by morning his sleeping bag would be soaked, even though it was no longer raining. He pulled the top edge over his face and tried to sleep, but it hit him then, the reason he'd forgotten his tent was because he'd been showing Sandy the workings of his office and he'd totally forgotten. He sighed he must put the woman out of his mind! Yes, she was beautiful and had the best personality he'd ever known, but she'd be gone in three months. What was there in Vansville to keep her there after the job he needed her for was over? Why should she stay during the winter when there was no work?

By the time Sandy lay down on her daybed for the night she was feeling very sorry for herself. Her stomach was growling so loud and so often she wasn't sure she could sleep through the noise. She'd drunk so much water she thought she might float away and that wasn't good, especially since she couldn't make fast trips to the bathroom.

The rain had tapered off as darkness fell and was a mist now, but she was sure the grocery store wasn't an all-nighter like they had so many of in Philadelphia. In fact, she wondered when it opened in the morning. Of course she hadn't asked, he'd hung up on her. She hoped it was before nine when she was to be at Ramon's. She sighed, it really didn't matter she had to get something to eat before she went to work. She would stay later at Ramon's to make up for any time she had to take to get groceries.

When she woke in the morning and looked at her clock, she debated when to get up. Finally, her stomach decided for her. She hurried to the bathroom, splashed her face and brushed her teeth, then drank a large glass of water, hoping that would keep her stomach from growling too loudly. She dressed comfortably and soon had herself in her van. She drove two blocks and parked in front of the grocery store, she had no competition the street was empty. Her spirits fell when she read the sign saying the hours were nine to five every day but Sunday. She shrugged, she'd stay later at Ramon's to make up for the time she spent buying her groceries and putting them away. She must have food to fill her stomach, shopping after work wasn't an option. She was glad for the Bible she kept in the van. Reading it would help her attitude.

It was eight forty-five when lights went on inside the store. The person opening the store must have a way to get in from the back, because no one had gone in the door in front where she was parked. At five minutes before nine, Sandy took herself to the controls inside her van and opened the door, then put down the lift to wheel herself on it. She lowered the lift to the sidewalk and wheeled herself off, then raised the lift and closed the door. By the time she reached the front door into the grocery, an older man was turning the lock inside. She wondered if this was the nameless man who had been so gruff with her yesterday. Never-the-less, she smiled at him. One always got farther with honey than vinegar, her mom always said.

He glanced at her, but didn't open the door for her. "Morning!" he called over his shoulder, as he moved away toward the back of the store.

Sandy leaned forward and pushed the door open, then wheeled herself inside. "Good morning!" she called back, immediately taking a cart. "I'm glad you open promptly, I'm a bit hungry this morning." She didn't continue the conversation or look at the man she was too hungry and wanted to get the job finished as quickly as possible.

Her voice finally registered. He'd expected a young woman to come in yesterday afternoon, but no one had, not even people he knew from town because it rained so hard. As Sandy began loading things into her cart, the man hurried behind the counter and slumped into a chair. He covered his face with his hands. He'd prided himself with taking care of the needs of this little town for the last five years, after he bought the store. It had taken one phone call yesterday afternoon to totally wipe his caring off the map. His conscience pricked him, big time.

About twenty minutes later the young lady pushed the cart up to the counter with one hand, while working the controls on her chair with the other and began to laboriously unload it onto the counter. He could tell that each layer would be harder for her to reach than the last. The man put his hand over hers when she placed a small package of meat on the counter.

When she looked up, he said, "Miss, let me unload that. If I'm not mistaken, you're the lady who called yesterday in the pouring down rain and wanted groceries delivered, aren't you?"

Nodding, she said, "Yes, I'm Sandy Bernard."

As the man came and began unloading her cart, he said, "I'm Alex Mallard. I'm terribly sorry for yesterday. From now on, you call when you need groceries, rain or shine and I'll have them there before supper. I'll bring them by as soon as I close the store. Will that work?"

"Yes, Mr. Mallard, that would be fine, bring the bill with you and I'll have the money ready. I appreciate your help now."

Sandy sat and watched, glad that he'd come to her rescue, she could throw things in, but she couldn't reach the bottom of the cart to get things out. The cart was unloaded and he pushed it out of the way. "I wouldn't mind if you called me Alex. I think we get in a rut sometimes and don't think too well outside the box. You know what I mean?" He smiled at her as he started running her things through. He hoped his smile dispelled any idea that he was putting her down. "Of course, if you'd whined a lot and said you was a cripple, I'd have listened."

She shook her head. "Alex, I've tried my whole life not to let this chair get in the way of being as normal as I can be. I would never have done that."

The man nodded. "I realize that, Ms. Bernard, now." Alex let out a sigh, "For five years I've prided myself on what a good job I've done for this town, but one phone call…"

Alex rang up the groceries and bagged them. Sandy looked at the screen and handed her money to the man. She smiled and said, "Alex, if you'll call me Sandy I'd really appreciate it. By the way, do you take checks? When you come with my groceries I may not have the exact change, but I could write you a check."

"Yes, Ms. Sandy, checks are fine." He looked at the huge pile of grocery bags and said, "Can I help you load these in your van?"

"I'd appreciate that a lot, thanks. Another question; yesterday Ted, Isabel's handyman, said I should put a sign in your window to advertise. You see, I teach piano and I'm wanting to get some students, if anyone in town would be interested."

Alex had been pushing the cart full of Sandy's groceries. He stopped dead in his tracks, turned fully around and stared at her. "You… you teach piano?"

"Yes, I have for several years and played piano for quite a few years."

He regrouped as quickly as he could and said, "Of course, Ms Sandy, you're welcome to put a notice in the window any time, just bring it by."

She smiled at him, as she opened the back door of the van and pulled out the first bag from the cart. "Thanks so much I really appreciate that. It's a bit hard for me to go door to door to drum up business, if you know what I mean."

Alex laughed. "I can imagine."

As Alex stuffed the last bag into the space, Sandy said, "I still have one more question for you, Alex. What can you tell me about that church across the street?"

"Sandy, I'm sorry to tell you I can't tell you much. My wife goes and nags me, so I go occasionally, but it's not for me – too loud."

Sandy smiled. What Ted said about this church must be true very few men went to it. So far, she'd forgotten to ask Isabel. Nothing they'd said when she arrived gave any idea if Isabel went to church, but Sandy had a feeling. She pushed the van's back door closed and said, "Thanks, Alex, for your help. I'll be by soon with a sign for your window. Of course, I need to get my piano here first. That's something I wasn't able to pack in my van when I moved."

Alex laughed. "I can imagine why! You have a good day and thanks for being so forgiving. I'm really sorry about yesterday."

She smiled and rubbed her tummy. "No lasting harm done Alex. See you!"

"Maybe so, but it's still unforgivable on my part, Ms. Sandy."

Sandy hurried back to her cabin, glad her stomach hadn't growled in the store. Back at her cabin, she let herself down, then went to the back and opened the door. She loaded her lap and the arms of her chair with as many of the bags as she could, making sure one of them was what she would eat now. Inside, she set all the bags on her table, then grabbed out the box with the cereal bars. She opened one and took a huge bite, then started putting away her food. After the first bar was gone, she opened another and took it with her to eat while she loaded up with more bags. It was after ten when finally she had her pantry, refrigerator and cupboards filled and her stomach had stopped growling.

Before she left for Ramon's, she went in the bathroom to relieve herself and splash more water on her face. She'd failed to turn on the air conditioner in the cabin before she left for the store and it was still warm in the cabin while she put away her groceries and the sweat was dripping off her chin by the time she finished.

On her way out she picked up the picture she had for him and put it on her lap to take with her. It was dry enough now to be hung and she would have it there for him. Inside the van, she placed it against the console and started up. She looked at her watch and sighed, she'd need to stay until one thirty to make up for the time she'd taken this morning. However, if he wasn't there it didn't matter.

When she arrived at Ramon's the same cars were in the parking lot and there were no lights on in the office. That only meant that the group he'd led hadn't chickened out in the awful weather they'd had yesterday. She put the picture back on her lap and let herself down onto the parking lot, then hurried to the office and let herself in.

She didn't see a spot where he would hang the picture, besides, she probably couldn't have reached it anyway, so she placed the picture on a chair. As she turned toward the desk, she noticed the red light on the answering machine was flashing, so she hurried behind the desk and located a pad to take down a message. After all, that was her job here in Vansville.

She hit the retrieval button and heard a dear, familiar voice say, "This message is for Sandy Bernard, this is her dad. Honey, I found this number on our phone bill and knew it was for the place in Georgia where you'd moved, so I'm calling. I know you haven't gotten your own phone yet. I've found a trucking company who will move your piano and treat it with kid gloves. They can have it on their truck on Monday if you can get me directions. They assured me they can get to Blairsville, but you'll have to supply the rest. Talk to you later, Sweetheart."

"Daddy!" she exclaimed. "That's great!"

Without waiting to see if there were any other messages, she immediately dialed and reversed the charges, but then she looked at her watch and before the call went through she hung up. Her dad wouldn't be there, only her mom. If there was a chance that she could get her daughter home and that was not to let her dad ship her piano, she'd do it. Instead, Sandy called the phone company and had the phone at her cabin changed to her own number. She wasn't happy she had to pay a large deposit, but that was life in the real world, so she accepted the bad news. It was after one thirty when Sandy closed up the office and headed to her cabin.

Over breakfast the next morning, Tom, the group leader said, "Ramon, what do we do with these wet tents?"

Ramon shrugged. "Leave them up until the last minute so that the sun can do some good. When we stop tonight, we'll pitch them first thing and open them up as much as possible. It'll keep the moisture from letting mold take over." He nodded toward his own sleeping bag slung over a low bush nearby. "As you can see, my sleeping bag suffered the same fate I'm hoping to get it as dry as possible before we break camp. Believe me, it's nasty sleeping in a wet bag."

Tom shuddered. "I'm sure that's true."

The sun shone brightly all day and warmed them. When it was time to set up camp, Ramon found a perfect spot. They were on the flat top of a high hill. In three directions was a breath-taking view. On the other side was a gurgling stream with forest beyond that. As soon as they stopped, several of the group dug out their cameras and began snapping pictures. What Sandy had said popped into Ramon's mind and he dug out his own camera. Carefully, he looked at each scene, judged the light and tried to take the best pictures he'd ever taken. This would be his gift to Sandy, a small thing in comparison to the picture she had for him. He could hardly wait to see it. *Umm, it's just the picture you want to see?* that little pest from his shoulder asked.

After supper, Tom said, "Ramon, did you say that Sandy was your new receptionist?"

"Yes, she came on Wednesday for an interview, so yesterday, when you folks came I was showing her my routine there at the office."

The man scowled and asked, "She came on Wednesday? With the line of work you do, why wouldn't she go on a trip first so she could be more acquainted with the area? Actually, I'd have expected to take her."

"I know she would if she could. She's an artist and she asked if there were places she could easily get to. Since she paints, I tried to be very careful when I took those pictures."

Tom scowled. "All the more reason. The views from this spot are awesome she should see them first hand."

"Believe me, she'd like to, I know."

"Why can't she?" Ginger asked.

"You didn't see that she sat in a wheelchair? She's paralyzed from her waist down."

"What!" another woman gasped. "She's what? No way! She can't be in a wheelchair, she's much too vivacious and positive."

Ramon nodded and bent over his backpack to put his camera away, hoping that no one noticed anything unusual about his expressions. "Yes, she's the most positive person I know, but she's permanently in a wheelchair."

Thinking back to the day before, Tom said, "Would she have left your office before the rain? Didn't you say she lives in one of those cabins I saw at the edge of town as we came in? Goodness, that's several blocks! Do you have taxi service?"

"No, we don't have taxis and she'd have been soaked if she stayed until after the rain came. If you noticed that blue van on my parking lot, that's hers. It is a slow process for her to get in it and I'm sure she would be soaked even before she was behind the wheel."

"Oh, my!" Ginger said, "I've never thought about what a handicapped person must go through. We take so many things for granted."

"Yes, we do," Ramon said.

By one thirty Sandy's stomach was growling again. She locked the office, having taken care of several voicemails and two phone calls. She was glad for the sunshine it was a relief from the dark, dismal day yesterday. She drove home and let herself in. After the bathroom, she headed for the kitchen and opened a can of chunky soup and ate it like a starving woman. After she cleaned up, she went to her closet and assembled her painting supplies, planning to drive somewhere and paint, but while she was there, someone knocked at the door. She put her paint case on her lap and backed out of the closet so she could answer. Before her stood Isabel.

Smiling, she said, "Isabel, what can I do for you?"

"Missy, the postman brought my mail, but then he said he had a letter for Miss Sandy Bernard and did I know her. I told him, of course, so after this he'll leave your mail here for you, but here's your letter today."

Sandy saw the perfect script her mom used and smiled as she took the letter. "Thanks, Isabel, it's from my mom. I'll read it in a bit." As she looked at Isabel, she had an inspiration. Isabel's salt and pepper hair was pulled back, but there were wisps of curls that had slipped out. She wore a colorful peasant skirt and matching top, she'd be a perfect subject. "Isabel, are you busy for a few hours?"

The older lady scowled and said, "Well, not really, why?"

"I'd like to paint your portrait."

"You...what did you say?"

"I want to paint your portrait," Sandy repeated.

"You want to paint *my* portrait, you want to put *my* picture on some... some..." she waved her hands around. "Some picture thing?"

Sandy smiled as she nodded. "Yes, Isabel. I want to paint a picture of you. You have the prettiest outfit on today it would look perfect on my canvas. Come on, bring a chair and come out to the porch. I know just where I want to do it."

"You can't be serious!"

"But I am, Isabel! Come on!" she said, enthusiastically. Sandy picked up her easel and took it out to the porch, then came back for the canvas, her pallet and brushes.

Finally, Isabel realized Sandy was serious and asked, "What chair do you want?"

"One of the kitchen chairs would be best." When Isabel brought it, Sandy showed her where to put it and how to sit. The porch was on the north side of the cabin, so there was never any direct sun, neither of them would have to look into the sun, but there was plenty of light and the background in the distance was awesome, it complemented Isabel perfectly. Isabel was a perfect model, she sat very still and Sandy had no trouble doing her painting. Finally, she said, "Okay, Isabel, you can get up now, I'm finished except for the background that I want to work on a little. Want to come see?"

Isabel nodded, left the chair and walked over beside Sandy, then stepped behind her to stand for a few minutes, looking at the portrait all the time. Finally, she turned and stood in front of her and looked Sandy in the eyes. Earnestly, she said, "Missy that is not me! That's some pretty old lady, maybe your mama you've painted."

Sandy laughed, shaking her head and curled her hand around Isabel's. "No, Isabel, my mom's pretty, but this is you. That outfit you have on is perfect for you that's why I wanted to paint you. Since you're standing there, turn around and see the background I plan to put behind you. Isn't that awesome?"

Isabel turned toward her painting and then faced the scene beyond the porch. "Oh, my! You will put that on that picture, too?"

"Yes! Won't it be wonderful?"

Isabel turned back around and looked at the picture, her eyes round with awe. After several minutes, she turned back to Sandy and extended her hands palms up, as if beseeching her, she said, "Could I have this when you're finished? I've never had anything like this done for me before." Looking into Sandy's eyes, with her hands still outstretched, she said, "I can't believe you did this!"

"Of course, Isabel, I planned to give it to you. It's like a house-warming present in reverse. I want you to have this. I'll get it finished this afternoon and it'll have to dry for a few days, but you can have it, say Monday or Tuesday."

"Oh, my! I can't believe it!" she whispered, in awe.

Sandy held her brush, intending to start the background the minute Isabel left, but she wasn't prepared for what Isabel did. Sandy held her pallet in her left hand and her brush in her right, but Isabel threw her arms around Sandy's neck and hugged her, kissing her on the cheek. Sandy immediately lowered her pallet and put her brush on the easel and put her arm around Isabel and kissed her back.

After a kiss on her cheek, Isabel exclaimed, "You are the sweetest person! I'm so glad you've come to be my closest neighbor."

"But Isabel, you're a great lady! I'm happy I can live so close to you."

Isabel finally left and Sandy grabbed her brush. The light was changing on the scene soon it wouldn't be as inspiring, so she quickly began her strokes to capture what she wanted. She breathed a sigh of relief forty-five minutes later when she finished. She took the painting inside and placed it beside the air conditioner so the air could dry it. She poured a glass of iced tea and took it back to the porch, intent on enjoying the last of the sun on the hills and clouds. When she had everything inside and put away, she fixed her supper and enjoyed it at her kitchen table. She'd left the chair on the porch, Isabel had taken it from where she planned to sit for her meals from now on and that place had to be open. She smiled, she knew without a doubt that she'd be happy in Vansville. She and Alex were fine and Isabel…well, Isabel was a treasure.

After cleaning up, she called home and gave her dad directions. She was excited when she hung up, they promised her piano would be here Tuesday. She couldn't wait to play some of her music perhaps tomorrow she'd make a sign for Alex's window and start her piano classes.

She didn't even hang up, but dialed 0 and Isabel picked up. "Hello?"

"Isabel, after you were here for all that time I thought of something I never asked you. Do you go to this church in town?"

"Missy, not that place! I tell you, that fella doesn't do as well as the Reader's Digest!"

"Really? Oh, dear."

"Are you serious about a church?"

"Yes, Isabel, I've asked everyone I've met in town."

"Then, you come with me on Sunday and I'll show you a real church." She took a minute as if she just thought of something. "But how do we do that?"

"The passenger seat in front is like any other van. You come ride with me and give directions and I'll provide the way."

"You want to go to Sunday school?"

"Of course, Isabel isn't that what going to church is all about?"

The older lady chuckled. "A girl after my own heart! I'll be at your van at eight fifteen on Sunday. Our Sunday school starts at nine and church is at ten. Our pastor says a lot, but he says it good and we'll be out close to eleven."

"Great, Isabel! I'm looking forward to it already."

"Missy, so am I! I haven't had company go with me to church in years!"

It was hard to get out of the dream. Groggy and disoriented, Ramon swam his way out of his sleeping bag on Sunday morning. The sun was already up and sweat was running down his face, as he pushed himself out of the bag. He couldn't quite remember what his dream was about, but he knew he had to get to the stream as soon as he could and splash water on his face. He pulled his feet under him and headed for the cool water of the lazy stream a few yards away.

Since he was barefoot and wore running shorts, he ran into the water until he was ankle deep in it then stood in the cool mountain water. After several minutes, he bent over and cupped his hands in the water and splashed his face, letting the water drip off his chin. They'd be getting back to Vansville today. He couldn't wait to get a razor onto the scrub on his face. On some of his trips he didn't mind the stubble, but today it felt awful and he wanted it gone.

Still with his feet in the water, he squatted down. His knees were bent and he laid his elbows on them. He looked out across the stream at the acres and acres of forest that lay beyond. He'd tramped those woods a time or two, but never taken a group into them, there were no trails that he knew about and he didn't take groups except on trails. He missed his solitary hikes he'd been so busy this year he hadn't been able to take any.

After sitting quietly in the cool water for several minutes, the self-appointed cook came to the stream with the coffee pot and filtering device. She filled the device with water and let it run into the coffee pot. She did it several times until her pot was full. Ramon watched her, but didn't say anything the lady didn't disturb him, either.

When the pot was full, she smiled at the handsome young man and said, "It's a beautiful day, isn't it? Since it's Sunday would you mind if we have a service before we start for home?"

Ramon shrugged. "I don't have a problem with it, Nancy. This is God's out-of-doors I just don't supply the music or the preaching."

Chuckling, Nancy said, "We'll sing a few songs, have prayer and read from the Bible. None of us is a preacher, but we do like to celebrate Sunday."

Ramon nodded and looked back at the forest. "That's fine, go right ahead."

"That's great! Ramon, you're welcome to join us. I'll have coffee perked in a few minutes and breakfast'll be ready soon."

"I'll wait for the aroma to call me."

Only moments later he was lost in his own thoughts again. Two weeks ago he'd had a group from some church in Atlanta who wanted to have a service on the day they'd get back. A few days ago, Sandy had asked about the church in town and he couldn't answer her. Today, Nancy asked if they could have a service. Church had never been part of his life. His mom never felt the need for anything but sleep on Sunday.

It had always been he and his mom until he was in high school, then she'd married Derek Casbah. The man hadn't made him very happy, but his mom seemed to be, but it hadn't changed his attitude toward church. Maybe some people needed that, but he didn't. He scowled, why did Sandy want to know about church? Was she into that kind of stuff? Why? Wasn't it God's fault that people were sick and handicapped? Why would she want to be associated with some god that did her wrong? He took a deep breath, then let it out and walked up the bank to roll up his sleeping bag, dress for the hike back home and load up his backpack. Well, make that after they'd had their little service.

"Breakfast's ready!" Nancy's voice sang out. "Come and get it!"

Ramon took his big tin cup and went to Nancy's coffee pot. As he poured, he said, "Smells good, Nancy. You've a way with breakfast."

Nancy laughed. "Young man, I've put meals on the table for thirty years. Tom and I've been married that long and we've had six kids, four of them boys. Making breakfast has been in my blood for a long time, believe me. I enjoy watching a man eat and in this great out-of-doors, breakfast is wonderful."

"Nancy!" Tom called out, "You've outdone yourself this morning! It must be you're anticipating getting back to the kids."

Nancy chuckled. "That's a possibility, Tom."

Ramon took the full plate Nancy handed him along with his coffee and went to his little camp stool that folded up to fit in his backpack. He sat on it and started to eat, but he noticed that most of those in the group bowed their heads before they took a mouthful. That other group from Atlanta did the same thing. Well, he didn't feel any need to bow his head he took his first mouthful and savored the flavors in the perfectly made omelet.

Watching the folks bow their heads first, then start eating made him think about Sandy. He hadn't seen her very much, but as one of the group said the other day, she was the most positive, up-beat person he'd ever encountered. He tried to think of a time when she wasn't smiling and he couldn't think of a time. Even when he knew she was unhappy because he'd told her he didn't need her at the interview, she'd smiled at him. It had been his undoing he knew he had to keep her, even if it was only for three months. He had to see her smile again.

Today was no different. He wished he didn't have a group coming at noon tomorrow. He'd see her for three short hours and most of that time he'd be distracted getting ready for the group he was leading. He sighed maybe he'd advertise in that same magazine and see if he could interest another guide to work with him next season. He looked down at his plate, it was still half full and the others were taking their eating utensils to the tub for washing. What was the matter with him? His eggs were nearly cold, so he shoveled several large mouthfuls into his mouth and washed them down with lukewarm coffee. When the last person dumped his things in the tub, Ramon jumped up. The rule was the last one done did the dishes. It was his turn.

"Ramon!" Tom exclaimed. "You finally get to do dishes! Were you daydreaming?"

Sheepishly, Ramon chuckled. "Yeah, guess I was." He smiled at the older man. "I'll do my turn at the dishes. That was a meal to die for!"

The lady who had fixed it smiled and said, "Thanks!"

FIVE

Ed knew it was the middle of the night, even though he still had his eyes closed. His room was dark, he could almost feel it. He opened his eyes, there was no light coming in the window because he had black shades he pulled each night, his door was closed he didn't like sounds disturbing his sleep, either. He looked at the numerals on his clock, the only light in his room it was one thirty in the morning. It was only his parents who slept downstairs and himself upstairs in the house, what had woken him?

He closed his eyes to pray, "Father in heaven, is there something You want me to know?"

The confrontation between his parents on Saturday morning came to his mind immediately. Sandy had called Friday evening and told their dad directions to the little burg where she now lived and he planned, after breakfast, to call the moving company with them. Colleen had literally raked him over the coals, telling him what she thought of his idea to send the piano. He'd never seen his mom so upset.

He sat up in bed, letting the sheet pool at his waist. "I must be here tomorrow morning and stay until the moving company leaves with that piano!"

They were scheduled to come at eight in the morning. If they did, he'd easily get to his ten o'clock class on time he only left right after breakfast to study in the library. Even if they were late, he could still afford to miss one day in that class. "Thank You, God! Thank You for giving me that message!" he exclaimed and fell back, asleep almost before his head hit his pillow. He slept soundly the rest of the night.

In the morning, Colleen was bustling around the kitchen before six o'clock, as she usually did, getting Charlie's breakfast so he could be out of the house by six forty-five. Before he finished eating, Ed wandered sleepily into the kitchen and slouched into his chair, his mom looked at him in surprise, he didn't usually appear before Charlie left for work. She poured him his wake-up cup of coffee and he grabbed it out of her hand.

After he took several sips of the hot brew, he turned to his dad and asked, "Dad, that moving company comes today, right?"

"Yes, Son, they promised me by eight o'clock."

"I have some things to do here, I'll be around." He winked at his dad.

Out of the corner of his eye he watched his mom as he said the words. She had turned back to the stove to dish him up a plate full of food. She held onto the plate, but the spatula, full of scrambled eggs clattered back into the frying pan, as she whirled around to glare at him. It was good the plate was still empty, food would have flown off she turned so fast. Neither man missed her action, even though she didn't speak.

Charlie nodded with a smile. "Great! I'm sure you'll be able to help them, especially with the cord and her little black pouch. Thanks for thinking of that, Son." His eyes said what his mouth wouldn't, or couldn't.

Ed took another sip of his coffee then said, "No problem, Dad. Did she take her sheet music, her metronome and all her other stuff with her?"

Charlie scowled, mentally thinking of her room. "No, I don't think so, Son. While you're waiting for the truck, could you check around her room and make sure all those things are packed up? If they'll take them, fine, if not, we'll ship them all another time."

Consciously avoiding looking at his mom, he said, "Sure, I'll make sure everything's ready in case they can take a box, too."

Colleen never spoke while her husband and son were talking. She quickly turned back to the stove, filled Ed's plate and brought it to the table. He knew she made a monumental effort not to slam it down in front of him. She went back to the stove and poured herself a cup of coffee, then came and sat in her place, making a great production of sitting.

Charlie looked across the table at her and said, "Love, aren't you eating with us?"

Ed saw her swallow before she opened her mouth, but she closed it again and swallowed again, before she said, "I'm not hungry yet, I'll eat later."

"It's such a good breakfast, my dear. I hope waiting until you're hungry won't spoil it."

"You're welcome," she said, between gritted teeth.

"So what's on for your day, my love?" he asked. "An outing with the sisters planned?"

Taking another sip, she said, "I didn't have anything special planned, just to be here when the movers came." What she didn't say out loud, but her eyes and body language said, was anything but cordial toward the movers. Ed said a silent *Thank You, Lord.* Colleen refused to look at her son.

Charlie chuckled. "I'll bet there'll be dust to clean up when the piano's gone."

"Mmm, probably will," she muttered.

Only a few minutes later, Charlie grabbed his postman's cap off the hook by the back door and placed it on his head. Colleen had come up behind him, as she usually did, but before she let him take her in his arms for a kiss, she hissed, "Did you tell Ed he needed to be here?"

Charlie put his hands on her upper arms, looking genuinely shocked. "Why no!"

Her eyes narrowed. "I thought you might have."

He shook his head. "No, I never thought to." He pulled her into his arms, noticing the resistance she gave him. "You have a good day, okay?"

"Mmm," she muttered.

He knew he couldn't stay longer, he'd be late for work, but he wished he could clear up the problem before he left. However, he knew this was not a problem that could be solved in a minute or two it had been growing insidiously for over twenty-five years. He wished he knew how to stop this thing it was almost like a cancer that was eating his wife up.

He eased her face up with his finger curled under her chin. Just before his lips claimed hers, he whispered, "I love you, Colleen, with all my heart. I'll see you this afternoon."

After their kiss, she pushed away from him and took a step back. "Yes," she said. Charlie picked up his lunchbox and headed out the back door.

Ed finished his breakfast, then found a large box and took it in Sandy's room. There were several things she hadn't taken that he knew if she was staying she'd want. He knew where she kept her music books, those she taught from and those she played from, so he loaded them all in the box and had wide tape around all the edges before he heard the truck out on the driveway. Quickly, he printed Sandy's address on the box with indelible marker. The front door bell rang and Ed ran down the hallway to answer. He wasn't surprised when his mom stayed in the kitchen washing dishes, not making a move toward the sound. The way his mom had acted at breakfast, he was sure she had planned not to answer the door at all when the truck came. Again he thanked God silently for waking him up last night.

Ed threw the door open and the man looked at his clipboard and said, "Bernard residence? A piano to go?"

"Yes," Ed said, "I think it would be easier if you backed your truck to the back door. We have a ramp to the driveway that you can wheel it down."

"Good, we'll do that first."

Ed smiled. "I'll have the door open for you."

The man smiled. "Much obliged."

Ed hurried through the house and in the kitchen Colleen blocked his way. "You're letting those men take the one thing that would bring her back!"

"Mom, we'll talk later. Right now, they need my help I'm sure they're on a schedule and plan to have her piano in Georgia tomorrow." Much to her surprise, Ed put his hands on her arms, lifted her off the floor and set her down a few feet away, out of the men's path.

Outside, the truck blocked the light coming into the kitchen. It stopped, but then a lift on the back whined as it lowered to the ground. A man stepped on the lift and opened the two long doors, then reached into the back of the truck. He pulled something and soon a dolly bounced onto the lift beside him. He and another man came up the ramp and Ed met them at the door.

"It's right this way, folks."

Colleen was still in the exact spot where her son had placed her and both men nodded to her as they went by. She never acknowledged either of them, but held a dishtowel and was wringing it into a tight knot. The man with the dolly went first then the other closed the door behind him. They followed Ed through the kitchen and living room into Sandy's conservatory. Colleen immediately came unstuck from the floor and followed on the heels of the second man. She stood silently in the doorway as the men moved the piano away from the wall.

"I'm sure my dad forgot to mention that we needed to send some small things to her. I have this box all taped up and her address on it, can you take it along with the piano or do we need to send it another way?"

The boss looked at the box beside Ed and shook his head. "No problem, we'll load them together and deliver them together. You got that taped up good, it'll do fine."

"Great!"

Silently, Colleen watched every move the men made. Ed could see she was seething it almost looked like smoke coming off her head. Her lips were in a straight line, her hands fisted tightly around the towel she was kneading that looked like homemade bread. She'd planted herself directly in the center of the doorway leading to the kitchen. Ed wondered if she would try to keep the piano from leaving the room.

The men strapped the piano securely to the dolly, one man tipped it back and the other moved to the other side to make sure it never moved. Ed grabbed up the box he'd filled and the men began to move, but Colleen didn't. Of course, Ed was attune to Colleen, so he moved quickly in-between the man backing up and his mom.

As pleasantly as possible, Ed said, "Move, Mom, that thing is heavy and you wouldn't want them to harm it in anyway, would you?"

"You!" she hissed.

The man was about to crowd Ed's back, as he took a step toward his mom, with the box in front of him. She either had to move or be mowed down by the box, her son, the man pulling the dolly holding the piano. She felt the box on her fists and finally realized there was nothing she could do to stop the inevitable. Finally, with it pushing harder on her hands, she stepped back and out of the way. Ed went first, opening the back door when he reached it so that the men didn't have to stop until they had the piano on the lift. They set the piano upright, then raised the lift with them both on it to the floor of the truck, then disappeared inside with the box and the piano.

Only a few minutes later, the men stepped off the lift, closed the doors and raised the lift. Ed signed their papers the boss took the clipboard and ripped off a copy of what he had signed. As the man handed the copy to Ed, he looked up and saw his mom standing at a kitchen window, he knew she was furious. Fortunately, the men didn't see her as each went to opposite sides of the truck, two doors slammed and the truck began to pull away. Ed sighed he wasn't looking forward to the confrontation that awaited him in the house. Why couldn't she let Sandy go?

Reluctantly, he walked up the ramp to the back door. Colleen wasn't there when he opened it, the bathroom door wasn't closed. He walked into the kitchen, but barely through the doorway, before his mom was in his face. "How could you do this to me?" she screamed.

Ed held up his hand and took another step, almost running into an immovable object that was his mother. "Sorry, Mom, I must get my things ready to leave for school. Those guys came pretty promptly, but I do have some work to do in the library for my second class. We can probably all discuss this when Dad and I are both here this evening after supper."

"You… you are…"

From the hallway below the staircase he called back, "Yes, I know, Mom, I'm totally responsible for the independence of my twenty-five year old sister."

"Oh!" Colleen muttered and collapsed into her chair at the table. She still held the wrinkled towel in her hands. When she realized it, she flung it to the floor. A few minutes later, Ed took the coward's way by silently slipping down the stairs and going out the front door. It was the long way to get his car in the garage at the back of the house.

Ramon had washed his clothes and dried them before going to bed Sunday night. He was up early packing while he ate breakfast Monday morning. He'd quickly checked his desk after his group left yesterday and admired Sandy's neat handwriting on his blotter and in the appointment book. He'd found the picture she'd painted and hung it in a prominent place in his office. Every one of the hikers had raved about the awesome picture she'd done.

He rinsed his breakfast dishes and filled his mug with the rest of the coffee he'd fixed and went to the office. This time, he'd already tied his one man tent onto the bottom of his backpack, it was the time of year when the mosquitoes were coming on in full attack mode and sleeping out among them wasn't something he loved to do.

He kept looking at the clock positioned on his desk and wondered at first why that was, besides, this group wasn't to come until noon. He'd been taking groups out on hikes and camping all summer, this group was no different, but he felt different. Then it hit him, in twenty minutes a light blue van was destined to come on the parking lot and a perfectly beautiful woman would leave that van and come though that door smiling for him.

"DeLord," he muttered, "get a grip! So she's a beautiful woman! Her job here'll be done by the end of October, why shouldn't she go back to Philadelphia?" Of course she would! She had a place to sell her paintings, she had students to teach. She didn't even have a piano here. He scowled. How did she play that piano, anyway?

However, in nineteen minutes a light blue van turned from the road onto his parking lot and his heart skipped. As he'd done the first time that van appeared, he watched the whole procedure. He realized that his heart pounded a little harder as he glimpsed the lady as she wheeled herself onto the lift. It was good his door was solid wood it gave him a chance to lower his head and pretend to be looking at something on his desk as she came through the doorway.

"Hi!" she said, enthusiastically.

"Hi, yourself! How's everything?"

She shrugged. "Last I checked everything's great! You made it back safe and sound?"

"Yes, even though it didn't start out very nice. We'd hardly gotten out of town before the clouds opened up."

"Yeah, I know. As it kept raining I wondered if they'd chicken out and return, but everything was as I left it when I came back the next morning, so I decided they hadn't. It was nice after that."

She wheeled herself close to the desk and asked, "Did you call your mom?"

He'd gotten the note she'd left him, he'd called Stew but not his mom. He made a face at her and said, "No. I don't always call her every time I'm back."

"She was pretty insistent. She said you hadn't talked but a minute the last time you called." Sandy made a face. "I totally embarrassed myself, I called her Mrs. DeLord and she informed me instantly that was *not* her name."

"No, she wouldn't even keep it before she got married again, she took her maiden name back, but she left me with the name."

"You don't like it?"

Ramon shrugged and said, "I didn't at the time, but I've reconciled with it now. So how's it been working out?"

With another broad smile, she said, "It's great, Ramon! I did as you said and penciled in some trips for November and one at Christmas time for an overnight to one of those shelters you spoke about. Several people who have been with you this year called and wanted to set up another trip next year. I penciled them in at the back of your appointment book, since you didn't show me one for next year, but I told each one we'd get back with them one way or the other."

Ramon was hardly hearing the words she said, instead, he watched her eyes, how they sparkled and pulled him in. If he'd been a fish, he'd be secure in her net already. "Were you planning on hiring another guide someday?"

"What? Oh, another guide? Yes, it was on my agenda for next year."

"Friday, just before I left, a man called who said he was Duncan Roads. He wanted to apply for a guide job and wanted to know if you had any more trips scheduled and if he might go with you on one or two of them. I told him you'd call around ten this morning, I couldn't answer his questions."

"This year?" Sandy nodded. "How could he possibly know that I wanted to hire another guide for next year?"

Sandy shrugged. "Maybe the Lord knew you needed some help."

Making a disgusted noise in his throat, he waved his hand back and forth, as if to wipe her statement away. He looked at her intensely and said, "Mmm, I'm sure. Sandy, this Lord of yours is no friend of mine. I never met Him I have no use for such as He, so I don't expect Him to help me out before I even need any help."

Sandy reached over and placed her hand on his. "Ramon, don't make any claims you can't back up. There is a verse of scripture that says, 'Before they call I will answer, while they are yet speaking I will hear.' Ramon, call the man, it can't hurt to have him go along with you. Surely he could be of some help, even if he doesn't know the area."

Reluctantly, Ramon agreed. He realized he'd either have to hire someone local who knew the area and he knew of no one who was interested or he'd have to hire someone from outside the area and they'd have to go along for several trips before he felt comfortable enough to send them out alone. Doing it this year would give them both a jump start for next year.

Ramon looked at the clock and realized that very soon his next group would be gathering. So far, only her van and his truck were on the parking lot. He said to Sandy, "I'll go in the house and make that call. The hikers will be coming soon perhaps you can entertain them for a few minutes until I finish talking to this man, Duncan."

She smiled at him. "Sure, I'll do what I can." Ramon stood up, grabbed the paper Sandy handed him and headed for the kitchen. He made a face, knowing that Sandy would do an excellent job of entertaining anyone with her bubbly personality. That lady was the world's best optimist. And he? Not so much!

When Duncan picked up the phone and spoke, Ramon almost felt jealous, even without seeing him. The man had a very pleasing baritone voice, one Ramon was sure would spark any woman's fancy. He was sure Sandy was not immune, why else was she so insistent on Ramon calling him right away? Probably because she wanted to hear the voice again and see the man who went with it. Of course, he couldn't come that day, but he and Ramon decided that he'd come over the Labor Day weekend, there was a three day trip and Duncan would join them.

Ramon walked back into the office as a large van drove onto his parking lot. "So, will he be coming?" Sandy asked.

Feeling that jealousy rear its ugly head again, he said, "Yes, he'll be here for my Labor Day trip. It's for those three days, I've taken those guys on hikes before and it's a rather hard hike. He said he's up to a challenge."

"Good, I'm glad you'll get some help. It seems to me, with only one day or as it is this time, only half a day between trips you're burning the candle at both ends. After a while, those ends meet in the middle and snuff each other out. Ramon, have you done this all summer?"

Sighing, he said, "Yeah, it's getting a little old, but that's why I hired you, I was getting behind in my paperwork."

"It didn't occur to you that you needed some help in the field?"

"Yeah. That's why I figured I'd get another guide next year."

Speaking reasonably, but not talking down to him, she said, "Ramon, if you train him this year, he can start off helping you next year."

All the passenger doors opened on the van stopped on the parking lot and six people climbed out, laughing and slapping each other. Before they came inside, they opened the back cargo doors and pulled out huge backpacks and leaned them against the van. The three men reached back and brought out three long items, two of the men laid one each beside their backpacks, the other tied his on top of another pack.

"What are they doing?"

"Those are two man sleeping tents. It's three couples going together. I warned them that evening and night time this time of year is great mosquito weather. It's okay until the fire dies."

"Did you take one last time?"

Ramon made a face. "I forgot mine, I got a little wet sleeping under the trees our first night, but I have it tied on already now."

"That's good. I see you hung your picture."

"Yes, every one of my group last time thought it was awesome! If you have any more and want to make a gallery out of this place, feel free. I'd be happy to let you sell them from here. Have you done any more?"

"I did one the other day of Isabel, but I gave it to her as a reverse house-warming gift."

"You gave it to her?" Ramon gasped.

Acting very nonchalant, Sandy shrugged as if it was a normal thing. "Yes, she's letting me go with her to church every Sunday now and she got Ted to fix that shower seat the same day. Besides, she came and brought my mail that day and she was dressed in a peasant outfit, she was perfect for a portrait."

Ramon shook his head. "I truly don't understand you."

Sandy laughed, as the first couple opened the door. "Does a man understand a woman?"

The man answered instead of Ramon. "Absolutely not! There is no way to understand a woman. Their thoughts and ways are past finding out. Any man who tries needs his head examined! And that's the truth!"

Sandy gave him a stern look. "Thanks a lot!"

The man chuckled. "You're welcome, I'm sure." He held out his hand and said, "I'm Silas National, pleased to meet you."

Sandy held out her hand. "I'm Sandy Bernard, Ramon's new receptionist."

"Good, he's a bright man, after all."

With the silence after the movers left, Colleen seethed all day and by three o'clock she had gained herself a massive headache. When Charlie came home there was no good smell of supper cooking, the lights weren't on and all was quiet. He put his lunch pail on the counter as usual and went through the house to find her. Colleen's car was still in the garage, so she was either here or out with one of her sisters. He found her on the bed with a pillow over her head. He tiptoed in the room, changed his clothes and she still hadn't moved. He went to her side of the bed and lifted the pillow, but without opening her eyes, she grabbed for it, wanting to keep it in place. Charlie kept hold of it, then sat down on the bed in the little pocket she made with her legs bent up toward her chest.

"Honey, I'm home." he said quietly. "I think Ed'll be home soon, should you be getting up to fix our dinner soon?"

Not opening her eyes, she grumbled, "No, I'm not getting supper tonight. Leave me alone, I have a headache."

Looking tenderly at his wife, he ran his fingers through her hair at her temple and said, "It couldn't be because there's a dusty spot in the middle room, could it?"

She raised up so fast Charlie almost tumbled off. Her eyes blazed and venom spewed out, as she screamed, "I hate you both! You've made it so my baby won't come home, ever!"

Charlie set the pillow aside, then trying to take her in his arms, but having to fend off her fists instead, Charlie said, "Now Colleen, you know that's not true at all! Sandy is no baby she is our oldest child and very much an adult. She has been trying for years not to be dependent and has been thwarted at each turn. No, Ed and I've not been doing any such thing. We've only done what she's asked us to do to help her. We have and wished her Godspeed." His heart palpitating, he took a deep breath and added, "Sweetheart, I really don't think you mean it when you said you hate us both."

She sank back on the bed, grabbed the pillow that Charlie had laid aside and just before she plastered it over her face, she mumbled, "You can't love her like I do."

Charlie spoke softly enough that Colleen probably couldn't hear, "No, I can only love her as her dad and Ed only as her brother. Neither of us loves her like her mother."

For a few minutes he watched his wife. When she didn't move, he left, closing the door. He went to the kitchen and looked in the refrigerator. There was a big pot of chili Colleen had made two days ago. He pulled it out and put it on the stove. He could at least turn the fire on under the pot and warm up something for Ed and him to eat. He turned the heat on low then went downstairs to work in his shop until Ed came home. He wouldn't appear for several hours.

Charlie picked up his jigsaw and asked himself the sixty-four million dollar question. Why was Colleen stuck on Sandy being an invalid and needing to be kept at home? Did she not feel useful now that all her children had left? He loved her, he needed her, oh, boy did he need her! He started cutting out an object he had in mind to make for Marcy's birthday that was coming in a little over a week. He loved working with his wood it gave him time to think.

Ed was not quiet when he came inside, so Charlie laid down his saw and went upstairs. From the cellar door, he looked at his son and said, "Maybe you should be a little more quiet, Son, your mom has a headache."

Ed made a face. "I'm sure she does. She was about to give me what for this morning, but I walked out as soon as I got my things together after the truck left. Unless she called and talked to one of her sisters, she's bottled it all up inside." Ed slung his books on the wide windowsill and asked, "Dad, why is she doing this to herself? I didn't really want Sis to go so far away, but I understand completely."

Charlie shook his head. "I have no idea, Ed, unless it's the empty nest syndrome. I'm told that's quite important to a woman, especially a stay-at-home mom."

As a typical college student, Ed slouched into a chair and said, "I've heard that. She's been really bad about Sandy. Marcy's her baby and she didn't make a peep when she went to nursing school. She's rarely home and I'm home every night."

"I don't know, Son. It's got me baffled, too."

Ed raised his head and sniffed. "What smells good?"

"Your mama's chili. I pulled the leftovers out of the fridge and it's heating on the stove. Mama told me she's not fixing supper for us."

Ed immediately dug his keys from his pocket and said, "I'll run down to the market and get some French bread to go with it!"

"Great! That'll go perfectly, Son. Thanks for thinking about that. Mama always has some kind of bread with chili, but I never thought about it."

By the time Ed went to his room for the night, Charlie had gone in their room and closed the door. Colleen hadn't come out, so she had conveniently bypassed any discussion about her feelings with her family. Charlie, turned on the dim light on his side of the bed, then undressed and crawled into bed. Colleen hadn't moved when he turned out the light. He sighed he'd never realized how much she hated change and conflict. Hadn't she been watching her children grow up, especially Sandy? Charlie was tired, he had a long walking route, so when his head hit the pillow it wasn't long before he was asleep.

Colleen waited until she knew Charlie was asleep then she got up and stalked from the room in her stocking feet. She hadn't undressed when she lay down with her headache. She went to the kitchen and was dumbfounded to find it clean and swept the men had taken care of their supper mess. She hadn't gone to the bathroom off their room, she didn't want to wake Charlie, but she went to the little room beyond the kitchen. She turned on the bright light and looked at herself in the mirror over the sink and saw the ugly lines her headache had caused. She splashed her face with cold water, hoping to erase at least some.

Moments later she left the bathroom and went to Sandy's conservatory, that couldn't be called that, since nothing of hers was there. She sat on the daybed and stared at the empty spot where the piano had been for so many years. Just as Charlie said, there were dust bunnies in the bare space. She'd refused to enter the room all day, so the dust was still on the wall where the piano had been. She must clean in here tomorrow. Just to spite him… no she wouldn't.

Angrily, she looked around the room. Sandy had taken everything she could fit into her van when she left. Today, everything else had gone in a box and been taken with the piano. Now it was just a room in the house she shared with Charlie and Ed. Of course, they had her pictures scattered throughout the house and there were three still hanging in this room, but that was all there was of her daughter. Her *cripple* daughter. How could she let herself be seen out in public? Colleen had been mortified for years each time Sandy wanted to go out in public. She'd even tried to disguise her chair when Sandy had played the recital at their church. Sandy wouldn't let her.

Twenty-five years ago the pastor and deacons had prayed for her, they'd anointed her with oil, but God hadn't healed her. She and Charlie took her to two brilliant neurosurgeons, but they couldn't do anything, her spinal cord had been severed in that nursery accident and would never give feeling below her waist, the damage was permanent, a spinal cord never rejuvenated. Their baby would never walk. She'd tried to shield her, she shouldn't have to live through the stares that kids give someone who's different or the snubbing people give people who don't look or act like them. Why couldn't she, her dad and siblings understand how her mom felt?

She sighed, she'd slept for several hours and now she wasn't tired. Her headache was only a dull throb in her head now. Maybe she'd clean. She found her mop pail and filled it with warm, sudsy water, hardwood floors kept their shine better if they were washed. She didn't need to use the loud vacuum cleaner on a wooden floor. She could also use her damp mop on the wall to take off the dust.

Colleen went back to bed about one thirty. She slipped in very quietly, leaving the light off and climbed under the covers next to her husband. She didn't cuddle up to him, as she usually did, he was asleep and she was still very angry with him. She turned away from him and closed her eyes, willing herself to sleep. However, her body knew what time the alarm went off and she was awake before it sounded.

She scurried into the bathroom and brushed her teeth, then drew her robe around her. Charlie was at the door when she pushed it open. He smiled at her, bent down and kissed her nose. One side of her mouth turned up, that was all the smile she could muster. She fled to the kitchen and started the coffee. Surprising them this morning, Ed joined them before Charlie left.

"Hi," he grumbled. "Mom, you got coffee?"

She nodded and poured him his mug full. "Thanks," he said and slouched in his chair.

"You're up early two days in a row, Son, why?" Charlie asked and sipped his coffee.

"Dad, we didn't get to the bottom of anything yesterday. I think we need to have a family discussion about what happened here yesterday."

They both heard the hiss come from the stove area. Colleen couldn't get away from the kitchen this morning. "What's there to talk about?" she grumbled.

"Mom, you screamed at me yesterday after Sandy's piano left and said it was my fault. You told Dad you hated both of us. I think there're lots of things to talk about."

"Sweetheart, you don't hate us."

Colleen narrowed her eyes to almost slits, before she answered, "I am absolutely furious that you let her go in the first place and then to pander to her wishes and send her piano to some godforsaken place hundreds of miles away! Maybe I don't **hate** you, but I surely am really, really angry at what you've done!"

"Why?" Ed asked. "Besides, how do you know it's a godforsaken place?"

"Mama, she's twenty-five years old, she's been voting for seven years. She has a means of getting herself around by herself, both in a building and out in public. Why should we not let her be the adult she is?" Charlie asked.

"She's a *cripple!*" Colleen screamed. Why couldn't these men understand?

Ed's mug of coffee sloshed on the table as he slammed it down. He was off the chair in the same movement and was in his mother's face in one long step. "Mom! She is *not, **not**,* a cripple! She's a young woman with a handicap! She works with her body doing everything she can to be an independent adult just like everyone else. You left your father's home when you married Dad. Dad left the old country and his family to come here. He was younger than Sandy when he did. She has every right to live her life as she wants and where she wants."

Colleen had bent back in her chair, her back straight against the wooden back, her head thrown back so she could look at her son, but not have him in her face. She shook her head and whispered, "She's my baby!"

"NO!" Ed thundered and pounded his fist on the table close to his mom's mug of coffee. "She's not your baby! She's grown up into a beautiful young woman. She deserves the greatest amount of respect anyone can shower upon her. She could be a bitter woman she could have your attitude and hide in the house all the rest of her life. Instead, she's cultivated outside interests, she practically taught herself to paint because you tried to thwart her at every turn. She's a genius on the piano, but not because of your help. You never let her go to school, but she learned from our books and got better grades than either Marcy or I got. She's not a baby she's a grown woman who needs to be acknowledged for who and what she is."

Colleen sniffed, but didn't say anything. Charlie didn't speak either. Ed had said everything that needed to be said and that Colleen needed to hear. He had stopped eating when Ed vaulted from his chair. He picked up his fork and finished his breakfast, swallowed his last mouthful of coffee and stood up.

"I guess it's time for me to leave. I'll see you later."

Finally, Colleen spoke. "Charlie! Aren't you going to reprimand your son for speaking to me like he did?"

He looked at her kindly, but there was no smile on his face and his voice was stern. "No, Colleen, I'm not. He spoke only the truth he was not disrespectful to you. I'm glad our son stands up for his sister the way he does." He looked at Ed and said, "Thank you, Son, you spelled it out perfectly. I'll see you both tonight."

Ed slumped into his chair, picked up his fork, stuck it in his cold eggs and said, "Thanks, Dad." *Not that it matters,* he added silently. "Umm, have a good day I'll see you at supper. Don't work too hard."

Ed finished his cold breakfast, took his morning shower and dressed for school. He didn't say anything else to his mom as he went back through the kitchen and out the back door to the garage. Colleen was facing the sink with her hands in the dishwater when he went by. She never even acknowledged her son as he left for the day.

Not long after Ed left, Colleen saw movement outside the kitchen window. She glanced out again then heard steps on the ramp to the back door. Only minutes later, Marcy came through the door with a huge backpack on her back and pulling a rolling suitcase that seemed to be bursting at the seams. Marcy let go of the rolling suitcase beside the washer and struggled out of the backpack, as she said, "Hi, Mom! I had two days off, so I decided to come home. Besides," she sighed, "I need some clean clothes and the washers at school aren't like yours."

"I'm glad you're here, Marcy. Us women need to stick together."

Marcy scowled. "Sure! What do you mean?"

"It'll come clear later on, perhaps over supper."

Colleen didn't say anything else, so Marcy shrugged, then went back to the laundry room and started sorting clothes. She knew Colleen was still in the kitchen, so she called, "Mom, has Sandy sent for her piano yet?"

"It went out yesterday." Colleen came to the door of the kitchen, as she spoke.

"Great! Since she's gone and so's all her stuff, can I move in that room? You know I'm only here once every two weeks, it'd be lots easier."

Looking outraged, Colleen said, "Marcy! Of course not! Why, that's Sandy's room!"

"But why, Mom? So it *was* Sandy's room. When she comes back to visit, she'll need it and I can go back upstairs, but she won't be here much and I can use it."

Colleen's head was silently moving back and forth. "Marcy, she's only gone for a little while. She's coming back soon, I know she is."

Marcy pushed the knob on the washer so that it started filling with water. She put the lid down on her first load then went to her mom in the doorway. Realizing the problem, since they'd been over and over Colleen's attitude toward Sandy many times, she said, "Mom, she's taken a job in Georgia. She's emptied her room of all her things, including her paints. She's asked that you send her piano and you said it left yesterday. Mom, she wouldn't have done all that if she hadn't planned on living down there permanently."

Tears slid down Colleen's cheeks. She had nothing in her hands, so she wrung them together. Through her tears, she gasped, "No! No! She can't be gone! She must come back!"

Marcy laid a hand on her shoulder. She'd never known her parents to deny something so colossal before. She corrected that immediately, not her parents, her dad had always done the right thing toward Sandy it was her mom. As the older woman cried, Marcy put her other hand on her arm, then put them both around her and pulled her close. Colleen didn't resist, she put her arms around her youngest and cried on her shoulder. Great sobs wracked her body and Marcy's top was soon soaked. Finally, Colleen's sobs turned to hiccoughs and Marcy rubbed her back.

Quietly, in her mom's ear she said, "Mom, Sandy's told us she wants to be independent. When she was invited to Georgia to that interview, she took everything. She planned to stay there, whether she got the job or not. She's gone, she isn't coming back to live, only to visit."

"Why? I don't understand!"

"What don't you understand, Mom?"

Colleen pulled away, wringing her hands. "She's... she must be in that chair all the time! She goes out in public in that chair! She does that awful van thing. She... she rides that part up and down. She's no right to be on the streets with that. She can't... it can't be right she can't use her legs to drive it! People stare at her, they make fun of her they take advantage of her!"

Marcy knew she must say something, but she was sure it wouldn't make any difference, her mom's mind was made up. "Yes, she's paralyzed below her waist she must use a wheelchair to get around. But Mom, it's motorized, she can move it herself. The van is made especially for her, the manufacturer built it in such a way that it will work perfectly safely for someone who is unable to use her feet and legs. Do you know that people stare at her? Have you seen them? Have you heard people making fun of her? Do you know that people take advantage of her? Have you seen it happen?"

Fiercely, Colleen said, "I know it happens! She'll come home and mumble under her breath about someone or other and I know it's because they're making fun of her or taking advantage of her! I know it!"

"But Mom does that mean you want her to stay here in the house all the time? Mom, that's treating her like she's six or seven! She is not contagious! What she has is a disability, she couldn't even pass it on to a child!"

"Yes! Yes, of course! I want her to be here – here at home!"

Marcy shook her head. "Mom, what will you ever do if she falls in love with someone and wants to become his wife? Will you forbid them?"

Colleen's hiccoughs stopped immediately. Tear tracks were on her cheeks, but her eyes were clear and huge as she stared at her daughter. "Marcy, what are you saying!" she gasped. "Your sister would never marry anyone!"

Marcy shrugged she had never realized how colossal her mom's mind set was. "She could, Mom. She has feelings, she could fall in love. A good man could love her and ask her to marry him. If she's in Georgia, how would you stop her?"

"I… I'd go there and demand he take it back!"

Marcy looked her mom straight in the eye and said, just as vehemently, "No, you wouldn't, Mom! Dad, Ed and I wouldn't let you!"

SIX

Tuesday morning, before she left for Ramon's, Sandy called Isabel and asked for Ted's number. When she had it, she called him and said, "Ted, this is Sandy from Isabel's first cabin. Are you free after lunch today?"

"Sure, I'm free, what do you need, Ms. Sandy?"

Sandy's smile was obvious, even to Ted, when she said, "I talked with my dad the other day and my piano's to come this afternoon. I'm looking around this sitting room and know where I want to put it, but I'll need to move some things before it gets here. It's a bit tough for me to push things and move my controls at the same time."

Without any hesitation, Ted asked, "You get off at noon, don't you?"

"Yes, I think if you could come about one o'clock that would be great."

"I'll be there, Ms. Sandy."

"Super! Thanks a lot, Ted."

Ted hung up shaking his head. That young woman was something else. She was the happiest, most vivacious, most energetic woman he'd ever met. She painted beautiful pictures in no time at all and now he learned that she played the piano. How could she do that? What more could she do? And all that while sitting in a wheelchair! He had never seen her legs move by themselves. They looked fairly normal, maybe a little small compared to the rest of her, but he'd never seen them move. What was it about her that was so different? Weren't most handicapped people angry or bitter?

Sandy hurried home from Ramon's and fixed a sandwich. At one o'clock, Ted knocked and Sandy let him in. She had her trademark, her lovely smile that he knew was genuine, in place as he walked through the door. She knew right where she wanted the piano and she had moved as much as she could out of the way and off the entertainment center, so it didn't take Ted long to move the small piece of furniture, the TV and stereo to a different part of the room, where she told him she wanted it. However, they were finished only seconds before they both heard a truck's brakes grind on the parking lot and heavy tires crunch the gravel.

Sandy looked out her window and said, "Oh, my! They're here already! I had no idea when they'd get here." Making a face, she said, "My van's totally in the way, but if I move it, I can't be here, since I can't travel on that gravel."

Ted shook his head. "Ms. Sandy, let them worry about it. It looks to me like they can work it just fine. They have a dolly to put the piano on then with two of them to bring it in, they'll manage perfectly. I'll go see if they need my help."

"Thanks, Ted," she sighed. "It's at times like this I feel so helpless."

Fiercely, Ted replied, "Don't you dare! You are one fantastic woman. You do way more than I'd ever expect."

"Thanks, Ted."

Ted went out and Sandy followed him to the porch. Ted came up to the truck, as one man put down the lift. He said, "Will you need any help?"

"I think we could manage a lot better if that van wasn't there."

Nodding toward the cabin, Ted said, "The lady in the wheelchair on the porch drives that van. She must have it so she doesn't have to go through the gravel."

The man squinted through the sunlight toward the porch and said, "It's a piano we brought here! Who is it that plays it?"

Ted nodded back at the porch. "That lady."

"No way!" the other man said, vehemently.

"I assure you she's the one. No one else lives there."

Both men were on the lift and the boss pushed the button on the controls to take them up to the floor level. "We'll get that piano there as best we can from here. Oh, you asked if you could help. We also brought a large box, could you carry it in for us?"

"Sure! I'll do that."

"Thanks, man, we appreciate that."

The men strapped the piano onto the dolly and wheeled it out onto the lift. One man held the dolly while the other pushed the box out. Very carefully they brought the piano from the lift across the gravel, around Sandy's van to the walk up to her porch. Ted trailed them with the box and Sandy's smile grew with each step the men took. Her smile was payment enough.

"Oh!" she exclaimed, clapping her hands, "I'm so happy to see you! You've done a fantastic job getting that here. What's in the box?"

"I have no idea, Ma'am, some young guy said this stuff was to come, so we brought it."

"My brother. Thanks. Wasn't my mother there?"

The boss's eyes twinkled, as he said, "You mean the female storm cloud who tried to block our way at each turn?" Sandy threw her head back and laughed.

Still chuckling, she said, "Yes, you described her perfectly. She's a bit opposed to my leaving. Come on in with my piano. Ted moved things out of the way for that." As she turned toward the door, she said, "I'm sure you'll be able to see the spot we have for it."

Sandy led the men through the door then held it open. When they had the piano in place where Sandy wanted it, one man said, "Ma'am, if you don't mind, could I ask something?"

"Sure!"

"Umm, it cost somebody quite a bit to send this from Philadelphia down here to this little burg. Ah, *you* play?"

She looked at him and gave him a big smile. As with most people who saw that smile, it was infectious. "Have you got a minute?"

The man with the dolly looked at his watch, as he wound the straps around it. "We're a bit ahead, we have a few minutes."

Sandy looked at Ted and said, "Ted, could you open that box and see if you can find a black pouch with some wires on it?"

Ted took his pocket knife and slit the wide tape holding the box closed. Pealing back the flaps, he didn't have to look far to find what she asked for. He held the pouch up and scowled as he looked at her. He'd never seen such a contraption before. Sandy held out her hand and said, "Please bring it over, Ted, and I'll give you guys a mini-concert right now. How'll that be?"

"Yes, Ma'am!" all three exclaimed.

Quickly, she hooked up the wires and placed the pouch on the back of her chair where she usually put it, then ran her fingers over the keys. She knew the piano needed tuning now that it had traveled, but not so much that they couldn't understand why she wanted her piano where she was. Without any music, she began to play one of her favorite pieces, losing herself in the music for a few minutes. When she lifted her fingers, four sets of hands were clapping.

One of the movers exclaimed, "That was amazing!"

She turned around to see that Isabel had joined them and was clapping along with the men. "Wow! That was great! You didn't use any music either!" Ted exclaimed.

"No, that's one of my favorites I've played it many times." She held out her hand to the driver and said, "Thanks for bringing that. I really appreciate it. You drive safely from here."

The man took her hand, then put his other around it and shook it warmly. "Ma'am, with a concert like that, we'll be set for the rest of the day. Thanks."

She smiled and followed them to the door. "I'm glad I could do that for you."

When she turned back, Ted and Isabel were still standing in the same spot. Isabel said, "Sandy, you must have cringed every time that lady put her hands on the keys there at Sunday school! You play so well, and she does so badly."

Sandy chuckled. "Maybe I'd better ask her on Sunday if she'd like to be my first student. Do you think she'd go for that?"

Isabel laughed. "No, but she should be!"

Ted looked at her and asked, "Have you put signs in the stores I suggested yet, Sandy?"

"No, I haven't, Ted. I thought I'd wait until the music box got here, at least, but I'll get them up right away. Thanks for reminding me."

"Well, you be about it, young lady!" he said, fiercely. "If I had a kid, you'd have your first student, believe me."

"Thanks, Ted I appreciate your vote of confidence."

"Well, make up a sign!" Isabel exclaimed. "I'll take it to the store now."

"I will, but it'll take an hour or so."

"Why?"

Sandy smiled at the lady. "Because, Isabel, I'm going to incorporate my advertisement into a painting, maybe I can get some other business, too. As I understand it, Ramon's job will be over at the end of October. I'll need to have something to tide me over the winter."

"Ted," Isabel turned to her handyman, "have you seen my new picture?"

"I guess not, Isabel, what picture?"

"Come on, I'll show you." Isabel turned on her heel and headed for the door with Ted close on her heels. Sandy's smile followed them.

As soon as the two people left, Sandy wheeled herself to the box that Ted had brought in. Her smile grew as she began taking things out of it, first came her metronome, her student books, all her sheet music and piano books. She put all those things on her lap and took them back to the piano and arranged them as she'd had them back in Philadelphia.

She chuckled, as she arranged her things. So Ed had stayed home until they'd come for the piano and her mom had been a female storm cloud. "Thank You, Lord! Thank You for having Ed there," she murmured. "I know You were in that, because I never thought about it and Dad didn't mention it either when we talked."

Her fingers itched to start playing, instead, she took two of the small canvases Ed had put on the bottom of the box and put them on the coffee table, then went to the closet and pulled out her paints and easel. When she was set up, she began with her water colors to make a quick picture then in lovely calligraphy, she wrote her ad. By the time she finished the second one, the first was dry and after she went to the bathroom, the second was dry. Smiling, she took them on her lap to her van. She let herself down at the grocery store and went in with one of her pictures. When Alex finished with his customer, he looked up and smiled.

Always happy to see the lovely lady and her smile, he said, "Hi, there, the lovely Ms. Sandy, what can I do for you? With all you bought the other day, you can't be out yet!"

Sandy laughed and said, "Alex, I'm here with my ad for piano students. My piano came today and I'm anxious to get started."

"Sure! We'll put it up in the window right now."

He obviously expected her to hand him a sheet of paper, because when she laid the canvas with its wooden frame in his hand, he had to quickly adjust his hand to take the extra weight that was more than a piece of paper would weigh. He looked down at what she had placed in his hand then looked up at her.

"Oh, my! This is an ad for you piano instructions?"

"Yes, Alex, can you put it in the window?"

"Of course, Sandy, but this is a beautiful picture! Where did you get it?"

"I painted it this afternoon."

"Wow! This afternoon? Wow!" He shook his head. "A lady of many talents, you are something else! What an addition to our town!"

As soon as Alex placed the canvas in his large front window, she left and went down the block to the other store in town, the hardware/gas station. She hadn't talked with anyone in this store, so she wasn't sure about the reception. She filled her gas tank then took her canvas into the store. Two people were at the register when she went in and another person walked in behind her. Unfortunately, he ignored her, walked around her chair and stepped in front of her.

Her canvas still on her lap, she rolled her chair up beside the man who had ignored her and said, "Excuse me, were you in a great hurry to pay for your gas and leave town?"

He looked at her then realized what he'd done and his face turned fiery red. He cleared his throat and said, "No, Ma'am, I guess I got in front of you, didn't I. I'm sorry."

"Yes, you did. By the way, I'm Sandy Bernard, I'm new in town and I'm hoping to start giving piano lessons from my home. Be sure to pass the word." She held up her canvas sign. "Anyone can reach me at this number."

"Sure, okay. I'll remember that." The man was clearly uncomfortable.

Sandy rolled up to the counter with some cash in her hand. As she laid the bills on the counter, she said, "I used pump three to get my gas, here's what I owe for it. Is the manager around that I could speak with him?"

The man behind the counter said, "I'm the manager, what do you want?" He didn't act very friendly and she wondered what reception she'd get for her sign.

"I have something to ask you, why don't you wait on this gentleman first? Surely there'll be a minute after he's finished."

Nearly dismissing her out of hand, he said, "Sure, hey Fred, how's it going?"

Still feeling uncomfortable for the way he'd treated Sandy, he said, "Okay, it seems. Can you put this on my account?"

The man scowled, then hit some keys on his register, but the drawer didn't open. He looked at the other man and said, "Now, Fred, your bill's getting up there, you'll need to pay up by the end of the month, you know."

"I'll do my best, Brad, thanks again." He walked away immediately.

Sandy moved back to the counter and slid her canvas in front of the man. She smiled at him and said, "I'm Sandy Bernard. I'm living at Isabel Isaacson's and Ted came by to fix something in my cabin. I told him I wanted to give piano lessons there and right away he said I should ask if I could put a notice in your window. I'm here to ask you if that would be all right."

The man scowled. Lots of times he'd put notices in his large window, that wasn't a problem, but this woman gave piano lessons? She was crippled, wasn't she? He could see the chair she sat in and she'd used it to move up to the counter twice. How could she give piano lessons, didn't you have to use your feet for something like that?

Sandy could see the unspoken questions in his eyes as he looked at her. She didn't say another word, only sat there looking at him with a smile on her face. After a few minutes, he asked, "You got the notice?" He didn't see any paper or anything. If it was something she'd ripped out of a notebook, he might give her some grief.

"Yes! This is it right here." Her smile stretched as she picked up the canvas and turned it so he could read it.

His scowl deepened. "But that's a painting!"

"Yes, so it is. I was sure you'd want something high quality to display in your window, so that's what I made for you."

He looked at her, a look of respect finally coming to his eyes. "You... you painted this to put in my window?"

"Yes. Will it be suitable?"

The man looked again at the lovely little painting then lifted it carefully off the counter, putting his hands along the sides, reading it as he walked toward the window. "It certainly will be! Sandy, you said your name is?"

"Yes, that's right. If someone asks, I'm usually home after twelve thirty each day. What was your name again?"

The man cleared some things out of the way then carefully placed the lovely picture in the window so that anyone coming in the store had to see it. He turned around and held out his hand, giving Sandy a ghost of a smile. "I'm Brad Thomas. I'm glad to make your acquaintance, Ms Bernard. I'll be sure to pass the word along." He dropped her hand and asked, "By the way, I don't mean to be rude, but how do you teach pi-ana?"

She grinned and moved her fingers out in front of her. "It's easy, beginners run their eight fingers and two thumbs up and down the keys like this."

He chuckled. "I guess I really wanna know how *you* play pi-ana. Oh, I know ya run your ten fingers up and down them keys, but isn't ther somethin' pi-ana players do with their feet?"

"Ahhh, now I understand what you're asking. Yes, most pianists do use their feet on the pedals, but you see, I have a special piano that does what it's supposed to without mine." She chuckled, turned toward the door and pushed it open. As she ran her chair over the threshold, she said, "Brad, you have a good day!"

He chuckled, as he watched the beautiful young woman take herself across the lot to her van, then up and inside. As the door closed, he said to himself. "That lady is somethin'! She never did tell me, so I don't know how she got crippled, but she sore don't let it get her down. That's the truth!" He shook his head. "She plays the pi-ana and can't even move her feet, amazing!" He'd been a little on the gruff side all afternoon, but she'd put a smile on his face.

Ramon was on the trail. He'd brought a group back Sunday evening and then this group came in Monday morning and left at noon. These people had booked their hike for four and a half days. They'd get back at dusk on Friday. He'd only had a few minutes with Sandy on Monday and it hadn't been enough, not enough at all. He hadn't been able to take his film in to get it developed because he hadn't used up the last two pictures, but before Wednesday he had a new roll in the camera. He couldn't wait to see the pictures that he'd taken with Sandy in mind.

On Monday, she'd talked nearly non-stop about getting her piano on Tuesday. He was trying to puzzle out how she could play the piano and have it sound like anything when her legs wouldn't move. His grandmother had played the piano after a fashion and she'd used her feet all the time. He knew Sandy couldn't use her feet, he had never seen them move, not ever. She always had them crossed at her ankles. She drove a van that was equipped for someone who couldn't use their legs. How could she play piano?

Later, Ramon felt like the odd man out. There were three couples sitting around the campfire snuggling together singing camp songs and roasting marshmallows, but Ramon sat alone. He sang and roasted marshmallows, but there wasn't anyone to put his arm around. It was the first time in a long time he felt his bachelorhood and tonight he didn't care for it.

One of the girls noticed he sat alone and asked, "Ramon, don't you have a girl friend?"

He shrugged. "I haven't felt the need, so, no, I don't have one. Besides, in my line of work I'm alone most of the time. I've never found a girl who shares my interest in hiking and backpacking. This whole summer I've only had a day or two off every week or so, that's not very promising for dating, do you think?"

"Really? You do this all summer long and only take a day or two off? Man, you must be really busy!" her husband exclaimed.

"This year I've been more busy than any year since I started doing this. I've toyed with the idea of hiring another guide, in fact, I talked with someone the other day who's interested and he's coming on the Labor Day hike. I'll see how it works out."

The girl's husband said, "So Sandy's not your girlfriend?"

"No, she came last week as my receptionist. She'll probably leave in October." *Your nose is growing, Pinocchio! Maybe she's not your girlfriend, but you'd sure like to make her the wife by your side.*

Another girl shook her head. "That painting she did for you is awesome! You say she did it at that pull-off down the road from Blairsville?"

"Yes, one afternoon. Actually, in only a few hours."

"I noticed she sat in a wheelchair, how does she get around? Does she have someone with her who drives her or something?"

Shaking his head, Ramon said, "That light blue van is hers. There's a lift in there that she operates so she can get in and drive."

"So all the controls are up where she can reach them with her hands?"

"Yes, I've never seen inside the van, but that has to be it, I've never seen her legs move. I've seen her readjust them with her hands a few times, but never on their own."

"If she paints so well, why's she working for you?"

Ramon shook his head. "Beats me! I have no idea. She told me she has her own gallery in Philadelphia and she's a piano teacher."

"Piano *teacher!*" several of them exclaimed. "How in the world ...? My mom play's for the church and she uses her feet all the time!" one man added.

"Yup. I haven't seen it, but that's what she's told me."

"Man alive! That's something else!"

Friday morning when they rolled up their tents and sleeping bags they had to hurry. The sky was dark and the clouds heavy. They hurried through their breakfast and pulled out their rain slickers from their backpacks and put them on before they hunched into their backpacks. Only a few minutes after they started down the trail back to Vansville the rain started. At first it was only a few drops, but an hour later it was coming down in earnest and the trail was getting muddy, which slowed them down. Ramon hadn't planned to get back before noon, but it would be much later than he'd planned, it would be close to supper time, maybe even close to dusk. This was the major drawback to hiking.

They weren't far from Vansville and he wondered how Sandy made out. She shouldn't be at the office when they arrived, but if she'd come, she'd left in the rain. Did she have anything to keep her dry? She'd be gone when he got there and his next hike started on Sunday, so he wouldn't see her at all. He sighed, seeing her smile was what he needed and he'd have to wait until Thursday before he could see it again. The thought crossed his mind that Isabel's cabins weren't that far away he could go see her - to see how work was going for her, of course.

One of the girls turned to ask, "Ramon, will Sandy be there when we get back? Does she stay at your place?"

"No, she won't be. She lives in one of the cabins up the road and she works from nine to twelve weekdays. She shouldn't be there, not with our getting back so close to supper."

"But I could come back some weekday morning and ask her about painting me a picture? Would that be all right?"

"Of course! That's one reason I hung her picture there in my office. I told her she could make a gallery out of it if she wanted and she said she'd consider it. Not too many people other than my hikers come there, but perhaps some who hike would like to buy a picture."

"I for one want one something like that one you have."

"She paints in oils?"

"She tells me she uses oils, watercolors and charcoal, so I guess she's pretty versatile. She told me the last time I saw her that she'd done a portrait of the lady whose cabin she lives in. I haven't seen it, though."

The youngest couple had only been married for a few months. She looked up at her husband, then at Ramon and said, "A portrait, I wonder if she could do one of us?"

Ramon shrugged. "I guess you'll have to ask her."

"Oh, we sure will!"

They were a bedraggled bunch when they finally came to the end of the trail on Ramon's parking lot. As he suspected, there was no blue van on the lot, but a light was shining through the window. He said goodbye to the three couples then went through the door into his office and was glad for the light that scattered the gloom from outside. He heard the van leave and he felt alone, more alone than he'd felt in a very long time and he wouldn't see her until Thursday.

There was a note on his desk. At least he could hold something she'd written. Did he have it bad, or what? It said, "Ramon, you're probably going to get back around supper time. If you're not too tired, come on over and share a home-cooked meal with me. If you'd like, I'll even play you a mini-concert after dinner. Sandy."

A grin spread across his face, the pack on his back felt like only a feather. Before he left the office, he shed his wet shoes and his pack, grabbed up his phone and dialed the number Sandy had added to the end of her note.

When she answered, he started grinning, even before he said, "Sandy, I got in and found your note. Is a half hour okay?"

"Of course, Ramon! I have spaghetti sauce simmering and I'll put the spaghetti on in a minute. Just bring yourself, oh, and dodge the raindrops!"

He laughed. "Sure! I'll see you soon."

He left his soaked hiking boots by the door, but took his backpack straight to the laundry. He emptied the large pocket with his clothes into the washer and started the machine. Quickly, he dumped out the other things and spread them out on the table. They weren't wet, but they felt damp. He stretched the backpack over the back of a chair so it could dry out.

As he left the laundry room, he began to shed his wet clothes and by the time he walked into the bathroom he was ready to step into the shower. He adjusted the temperature and was glad for the warm water. Washing up in cold stream water wasn't bad when the weather was warm and sunny, but a warm shower at the end of a very rainy day was most welcome. He washed his hair and felt a hundred percent better.

After a shave and some deodorant, he hurried into his bedroom and pulled on some clean underwear and socks, but then ground to a halt, wondering what to wear to Sandy's place. Should he consider this a date? Should he dress up? Was she feeding him because she felt he was special or because he'd come home in the rain? He shrugged, pulled out a pair of creased black jeans, his nicest pair of black shoes and a black silk shirt. He looked at his assortment of string ties, but shook his head and left them all on the rack. That was a little much, he decided.

It had been an impulse for Sandy when she was at the office. She'd come at nine and the rain hadn't started. She'd done her work, then found a blank piece of typing paper and done a charcoal of the hill she could see out the side window of the office. The clouds had hung low over the hill and she felt she'd captured the dismal day perfectly. Of course, it was raining when it was time to leave, so she'd slid the picture into a plastic file folder and slid it down between her back and the chair back. She'd been wet when she got to her cabin, but the picture wasn't.

It had also been an impulse to write that note to Ramon. She'd thought about it all morning. Every time she looked outside the rain was coming down, making the puddles grow. Several times the fog had blown in over the parking lot and she'd thought of the hikers out on the trail. She was sure Ramon had nothing planned for the evening other than washing his clothes and getting ready for his next hike, scheduled for Sunday.

Once she'd written the note she'd thought about tearing it up several times. What would he think of her asking him over to eat with her? After all, she was a single woman and he a single man. She didn't want to lead him on, but she always came back to the decision to offer a meal. Did he eat properly when he was home alone? Men were notorious for slapping something together, and not necessarily have it good nutrition.

After his call, she plopped the spaghetti into the boiling water, then hurried to her closet. She was mostly dressed, but she'd waited to put on her slacks and top until after she finished the sauce, in case she spilled something, it might burn her legs, but she wouldn't feel it and she'd keep her slacks clean. She was glad she hadn't spilled anything, but she did hurry into the rest of her clothes. A half hour wasn't too long. She pulled her blouse over her head and her tiny chime clock tinkled the time. She looked in the mirror over her bathroom sink, grabbed up her brush and swished it through her hair.

Ramon knocked on Sandy's door in half an hour. She was at her kitchen sink, so she called, "Come on in out of the rain!"

The wonderful aroma of homemade spaghetti sauce had reached him on the porch, so he pushed the door open and had his nose in the air. "What a terrific smell! You know exactly the way to a man's heart, or maybe it's his stomach."

Sandy chuckled. "Oh, come on, Ramon, spaghetti is spaghetti, you know."

He walked over to her at her sink and handed her a small bunch of wild flowers he'd rushed out into the rain to pick from his backyard. She looked up at him as his hand held the flowers and said, "Ramon! How beautiful! I'll rinse out this jar and put them in it. I don't have a vase, but we'll put them on the table." She looked him over and said, "Wow! You really look sharp! That outfit's a lot different from your hiking gear. This is nothing like hiking boots and khaki pants." Her eyes twinkled. "I wondered if you had anything else."

He chuckled. "You must remember I have five months I must dress myself in something else besides hiking gear."

"Of course, how could I forget that?" She smacked her hand on her forehead. "Of course! Five months, is it that long?"

"Can I do anything?"

"Not a thing, I must only rinse the spaghetti and then we'll eat. I poured you some iced tea. You drink that a lot at your place, so I figured that would be fine."

Ramon slouched onto the chair at the table where Sandy had set a place for him. Her place was obvious. "Tea's great. It's always good to be back to sit on something besides a camp stool or the ground. A chair with a back is a luxury." He saw her picture hanging over the toaster. It wasn't high, she must have hung it. "Sandy! Did you do this picture?"

"Does it look a bit familiar?"

He looked at it a little more closely. "Yeah, as a matter of fact. It's what I see out the side window of my office, only it's partly obscured by rain clouds."

She brought the spaghetti and set it on the table. "Yes, I was a bit bored this morning, so between phone calls I drew it. Besides, I decided I need something to spruce up the place, so I'll do some painting." She could tell Ramon was about to pick up the bowl from where she'd put it, so she put her hand over his wrist and said, "Would you mind if I said grace over the food?"

Remembering that the lady last Sunday on the trail had asked her husband to say 'grace' over their last meal, he shrugged and said, "No, it's okay." He felt her hand on his arm and wished she'd put it on his hand, he'd have taken her hand and held it. He swallowed a sigh. Did he have it bad, or what? Still, didn't people like her have something against people like him?

She bowed her head and said, "Father in heaven, I want to thank You for bringing Ramon and his hikers back safely again. Thank You for the rain that the ground needs and thank You for our food. Bless this evening, I pray. In Jesus name, amen."

Ramon had kept his eyes open, while Sandy had closed hers to pray. He rarely listened when someone prayed on the trail, but he'd wondered what kinds of things someone said in a prayer. He couldn't believe she'd prayed for him and thanked her God for keeping him safe. Was that something people who believed in God did?

Sandy pulled her hand from his arm and he immediately missed its warmth. To keep from grabbing it back, he picked up the bowl of spaghetti and took a large helping, then handed it to her and said, "I see your piano came. Was it Tuesday as you hoped?"

She put a much smaller amount of spaghetti on her own plate and said, "Yes, just after lunch. It needs tuning, since it was jarred around in the moving truck and over the gravel out there, but I can't get a man here to do that until next week, so if you don't want to hear it tonight, it's okay with me."

Shaking his head, he said, "No, Ma'am! I want to hear something you play tonight. Besides, you promised me a mini-concert after dinner." He grinned around a mouthful and said, "I'm not letting you off the hook that easily, young lady!"

She sighed, "You didn't forget, did you?"

He grinned at her. "Of course not, I'm much too young to be senile yet."

She wasn't surprised when he finished up all her spaghetti and sauce. After all, he'd been on a trail for five days. Usually, there was one good cook on a hike, or so he said, but there were only so many things anyone could cook over a fire. She never felt like she'd missed out on anything, but since she'd come to Vansville and watched Ramon and his groups leave on their hikes, she'd wondered what it was like to sleep in a tent and cook over an open fire.

Ramon helped her clear the table, then stayed and dried the dishes as she washed them. He noticed that the sink was lower than his at home and she could reach in it easily. She sighed, as she draped the dishcloth over the spigot and said, "I guess if you want to take a seat in my living room I'll play you that mini-concert."

He followed her from the kitchen into the sitting room and sat in the chair closest to the piano. "I'm fascinated to watch you. My grandma played her own version of piano, but I don't think it was anything like what you'll play."

She chuckled. "You never know. I'm pretty versatile."

Ramon watched as she pulled herself up to the piano, but before she put her fingers on the keys, she took a small black pouch from the music ledge and slid it over the top of the back of her chair. She moved her back around against it then moved the pouch a little. When she was satisfied with it, she opened a piece of sheet music and let her fingers glide over the keys. Only seconds later, Ramon was enthralled. Music from the radio couldn't compare with this.

Before she had finished, the door opened without a knock and Isabel walked in. She looked at Sandy's back, then at Ramon then stood with her back to the closed door. When Sandy finished playing, Ramon began to clap and so did Isabel. Sandy looked around and saw her standing there and exclaimed, "Isabel! You've come again!"

By now, Isabel had shed her rain slicker and hat and draped them over a kitchen chair. As she came back to the living room, she said, "Missy, I can hear you playing from my living room. It is so wonderful I must come over to hear it better. I hope you don't mind?"

Ramon wanted to answer that question, but he kept silent, he was sure his answer might not be exactly what Isabel wanted to hear.

If he wasn't mistaken, he'd thought about Sandy everyday of the hike. However, Sandy smiled and said, "It's fine, Isabel, I invited Ramon over for a hot meal after his hikers left. I figured they'd gotten totally soaked today and a home-cooked meal would taste good."

"Will you play more?" she asked, hopefully.

"Depends if Ramon can stand this out-of-tune piano."

He held up his hands and said, "Hey, it sounds great to me."

Sandy turned back to the piano and readjusted her pouch then she played another piece that was quite intricate and several pages long. When Sandy raised her hands, Isabel sighed and said, "Your playing didn't stop the rain and I'm expecting a call this evening, so I best go. You're wonderful, Missy, I could listen to you all day."

Sandy laughed. "Isabel, I'm sure you'd get bored after a while."

When the door closed behind Isabel, Ramon stood and came to stand behind Sandy. He looked at the music she'd been playing from and shook his head. "Man! How do you make that into the sounds that came from that piano! You must be exhausted when you finish making your fingers go that fast!"

"No," she shook her head. "The only time I was exhausted from playing piano was that time I gave a concert at our church. The pastor had asked me to provide music for an hour and a half, with a fifteen minute intermission. I did, but I never realized that the audience would ask for two encores!" She shook her head. "The whole thing stretched to two hours and I'd been nervous to start. I was happy to let my dad lift me from the chair and drive me home. I slept really late the next morning."

"Wow! Two hours of playing! That'd be something! So you've only done that once? Would you do it again?"

"I guess I could do it again."

Taking his eyes from the music to look at the lovely lady in front of him, he said, "You know, I had a thought. The man who calls himself the preacher at the church here in town hikes with me occasionally. I could ask if he'd let you play."

Sandy shrugged. "I suppose."

"Did you put up those signs Ted suggested you put up to give lessons?"

"Yes, Tuesday afternoon, but I haven't had that first call."

"Maybe if people in town heard you play it might help you get students."

Sandy nodded, thoughtfully. "You may have a point. I'd have to do a little brush up, but I think I could handle it sometime, maybe after Labor Day."

"I'll talk to Roger and get something in the works." Ramon stifled a yawn. "You know, my body tells me it's wanting to get in that soft bed pretty soon."

"I can believe that! I don't want to hold you from leaving I sure didn't have anything planned out. You have so little time at home, feel free."

Ramon heard the rain still striking the roof and asked, "Have you seen or heard a weather outlook the next few days? Of course, I haven't."

Sandy laughed. "You mean you don't carry your own TV so you can flip on the weather channel and the news at eleven o'clock each night?"

Ramon chuckled. "No, not really. The worst it's ever been was a woman with her backpack filled with her cosmetics."

"Cosmetics! On a trail? Good grief! The weather. Well, after this nice gentle rain all day today it's to clear up tonight and be partly sunny tomorrow. You could work in that back yard of yours tomorrow and pull out some of those weeds."

Shaking his head, Ramon sighed, "When I realized how many hikes I had scheduled this summer I gave up on that weed patch. Last year I had time to grow some of my own food and had a tiny flower patch, but it didn't happen this year. People started calling for hikes even early in the spring this year!"

Sandy nodded. "You definitely need to hire that Mr. Roads and train him well. Next year, split the hikes with him and let him shoulder some of the load. Being busy is good, but like I say, you're burning the candle at both ends, you're bound to burn out one of these days."

"I'd planned to run the mower over that weed patch tomorrow if it's not raining. In the afternoon would you like to go for a drive on some of the country roads around?"

Sandy's eyes sparkled. "Ramon, you can't know how much I'd love to do that! Could I pack a picnic lunch?"

"If tonight's meal was what you do in the kitchen, I won't turn you down, believe me!" He scowled. "It would be easier if I could drive, but I don't guess that could happen, could it?"

"Ramon, there are two ways that can happen. We can put the passenger seat from my van in the driver's place and I can sit in the empty spot it makes on the passenger side or this arm on this chair can be removed and I can transfer into a regular car. It's a bit impossible to take this chair in a regular car, but I can sit on the seat."

"But then you couldn't get out, if we couldn't take your chair."

"No, that's right."

"We'll use your van. I'm sure there'll be times you'll want to get out."

She grabbed his hand and smiled at him and Ramon felt the need to put braces on his legs. "Ramon, I'm absolutely thrilled that you suggested we go for a ride! I really want to become familiar with this area, especially since I'm going to be living here now. Thank you so much. What time should I be ready?"

"It'll take a bit to mow all that weedy stuff, let's say eleven for lunch and the afternoon. Will that work for you?"

"It'll be terrific! I'll be ready. Thanks for coming tonight, too. It's been great!"

Shaking his head in wonderment at this lady, Ramon said, "I'm the one who should say thanks to you, Sandy! I've had a great time and supper was fantastic. I'll see you tomorrow."

Sandy followed him to the door and watched him run through the rain to his truck. He waved as he opened his door and she waved back then closed her door as the light went out in his truck. She headed for the bathroom to brush her teeth before she made herself ready for bed. She smiled, she'd get to see some of the beautiful scenery finally something she'd wanted to do ever since she'd arrived. She sighed, she'd be able to spend the time with a man she had great respect for, as well.

SEVEN

Ramon turned on the wipers and sat staring at the cabin. He raced the engine then realized he hadn't taken the stick out of park. No, he wasn't rattled, he was tired. Well, maybe he was a little rattled. He'd spent the evening with a beautiful, vivacious, intelligent young woman, who had more talent in her little finger than most people had in their brains. He'd asked her to spend the afternoon with him tomorrow and he was excited. He had to admit, he was lost he'd lost his heart a few days ago to Sandy Bernard. When he was at last in his soft bed, he dreamed about that young woman.

But…. 'The best laid plans…'
Millie Casbah didn't know about Ramon's plans with Sandy when she stopped by early Saturday morning. Ramon was still in bed, he was exhausted when he arrived home from Sandy's, so he quickly put his clothes in the dryer and then went to bed, but during the night a dream had woken him. It wasn't just any dream he'd dreamed about one beautiful, happy, vivacious lady who sat in a wheelchair. Then again, some hours later he'd had another dream with the same woman, but this dream had him blushing and lying awake for quite a while.

He woke up to knocking at his front door. He scowled and looked at his clock, and realized immediately that he'd slept longer than he'd planned, but not so late that someone should be knocking at his door this early. He dragged his jeans on and threaded his fingers through his hair to make the tangled ends lie down. Barefoot and shirtless, he went to the door.

Warily, he looked through the filmy curtain on the window beside the door and saw his mom. He sighed and pulled open the door. "It's about time!" she exclaimed, without apology.

"Mom, good morning to you, too."

"Don't be smart with me, Son. Why are you just now getting up?"

He covered a yawn. "Because it's been nearly a week since I got to sleep in a bed. Why did you come by so early?"

The woman looked like a movie star ready to step before the camera or glide down the Way of Lights in Atlantic City. It didn't matter that it was Saturday morning she always spent hours at her dressing table. Her hair was in perfect position, like she'd just come from the hairdresser, even though he knew she hadn't. Her nails had just been done and he could see snatches of her toes, with polish to match her fingernails and also her lipstick. As usual, she wore a perfect outfit, one that complimented her makeup and her shoes also matched. For a change they were not spikes, but four inch platforms with three inch heels added to that, that made her nearly as tall as Ramon. *How can she lift her feel in something so heavy!*

Looking her son up and down, she brought her eyes back to his and said in a pouty voice, "I wanted you to take me to the mall in Blairsville."

Without hesitation, he shook his head and said, "Can't happen, Mom. I already have plans that I'm not breaking." He nodded to the parking lot where her lovely Jag sat. "Besides, you have a perfectly good set of wheels that you love to drive that can take you to the mall in Blairsville, or you have a husband who could do the honors."

"You don't want to spend time with me!" she accused. He could almost see her bottom lip jutting out like some teenager.

"No, Mom, that's not it, but you must remember that I'm a big boy now, I'm pushing twenty-seven and I don't live to do your every bidding as I once did."

"What are your plans? I'll go with you."

His heart nearly clogged his throat he wouldn't have his mom go anywhere he took Sandy. "Mom, you will *not* go with me! First of all, I'm mowing my weed patch that used to be a garden other years in the back yard. I'm sure, dressed like you are that you wouldn't want to push a mower around that lot. Secondly, I'm driving out in the country for the afternoon." He put up his hand. "No, the answer is no, you are not going along, no matter how 'lonely' you are. Go to the mall in Blairsville, I'm sure you'll find some real bargains that you can't live without."

She scowled at him. "Don't make fun of me, Ramon! After all, I'm your mother and you need to respect me."

"Mom, I respect you, but it would mean more to me if you and I had some interests in common. You know I don't like your husband much and he doesn't care for me, not even a little. You get all painted and primped every day of the week, hoping that he'll notice and do stuff with you. Last I checked it hasn't worked yet. No, Mom, I'm not taking you to Blairsville and no, you're not going anywhere with me."

Tears pooled in his mom's eyes, but of course, they wouldn't fall, they would ruin her eyeshadow, but Ramon looked at his watch. "I have to go, Mom, I'll be late for my appointment and I won't get my yard mowed first. You have a good day. By the way, I'm out of here tomorrow for most of the week with another group. I have things I must do for that, too." He couldn't think of anything, but surely there was something he had to do tomorrow to get ready. ...Ah, yes, his clothes were still in the dryer. He'd have to knock the mud off his tent before he could attach it to the bottom of his pack, too.

Millie stood up as tall as possible, ran her hands down her sides, straightening invisible wrinkles, then looked at the parking lot for Sandy's van, then she asked, "The cripple's here through the week?"

Ramon's eyes narrowed. He'd never known Sandy to get upset about anything, but if he was in her place, he'd hate someone calling him a 'cripple.' Tamping down his anger, he asked, "Didn't Sandy introduce herself?"

"You mean that woman?"

Showing his irritation a little, Ramon said, "*Sandy* is my receptionist. She works Monday through Friday in the mornings. She has a name, Mom and she has a handicap. I'd say she could run circles around you in anything you tried to do. Don't put her down,

Mom. She's the best thing that ever came to Vansville. I'll say that without hesitation."

"So you like her?" Millie sneered.

Trying very hard not to let his anger blow up in their faces, he said, "Like I say, she's the best thing that ever came to Vansville." Ramon took the edge of the door and began to close it. "Bye, Mom, I'm busy starting now and I don't have time to play word games. Thanks for stopping by." *but don't bother coming back again.* he said to himself.

As the door clicked closed, Ramon heard, "Well, I'll be, what an ingrate!"

"Mmm, yes, what an ingrate!" he muttered, and hurried back to his bedroom to wash up and dress for the day.

He raced to the kitchen and started coffee through his coffeemaker, then raced to brush his teeth. The kitchen clock told him he'd have to grab his coffee and take it with him to drink while he ran his mower around. Breakfast would have to be a granola bar on his way to Sandy's. The confrontation with his mom, piled on top of oversleeping had put him way behind. How did she always know when to be the most disruptive? She always came at the most inconvenient times. He shook his head, how could she say such awful things about Sandy? She didn't even know her! As high as the weeds were, he probably would have to get up early tomorrow to finish mowing. He sighed, went back to the kitchen and filled his mug. Only moments later he was pushing the power mower around the weed patch, wishing it was self-propelled.

Millie stomped as best she could back to her car. She wasn't used to these platform shoes, four inches off the ground, then the heels another three inches. However, she would not make a scene at her son's house, even though she'd like to torch the place sometimes, then she'd divorce Derek and Ramon would live with her. So he was pushing twenty-seven! He needed to respect his mother! She jerked open the driver's door on her Jag and threw herself into the driver's seat. She wanted to be seen with a good looking *young* man. If they went to Blairsville, no one would know he was her son. Mr. Casbah, was wearing on her nerves, but she couldn't find any reason to divorce him yet. But she would! One of these days…

Instead of going to Blairsville by herself, Millie thought about staying down the street and following Ramon to see what his plans were after he mowed his backyard. However, she started her car and drove out of Ramon's parking lot. She stopped by the store, remembering the list the housekeeper had given her and said they needed. As she crossed the sidewalk to the door, she saw the beautiful little painting in the window.

"Wow! That's beautiful!" she whispered.

She looked more closely and saw the picture that looked like the scene through Ramon's office window, but splashed across it was a piano and the words, "Do you long to play good music? Wish you could let it flow from your fingers? Call Sandy, she'll give you a good price and a good start on your dream." Under that, she saw a phone number she didn't know.

She stood for a minute then said out loud, "Didn't he say her name was Sandy or was it Cynthia? His 'receptionist' must be Cynthia, there's no way a *cripple* could teach piano!" She huffed out a sigh and reached for the door handle.

She walked in the store and Alex smiled. "Hi, Mrs. Casbah, you're around early this morning. Has your housekeeper got a list of things she needs?"

"Yes, I have several things to pick up." Thumbing her hand over her shoulder, she said, "We got a piano teacher in town now?"

The grocer smiled at the unsociable woman. "Yes, Sandy brought that in yesterday. She's something! I must admit. She whipped that painting up yesterday afternoon after her piano came from Philadelphia. I haven't heard her, but Isabel says she plays like an angel. You know anybody who wants to take lessons?"

Instantly angry because this was about somebody not herself and somebody she disliked, she exclaimed, "No, I don't! Here's my list, I have someplace I have to be this afternoon." She slapped the list down in front of Alex.

Alex grabbed the list, realizing he'd probably said way too much to this disagreeable woman. How Ramon could have turned out like he did with her as his mother was beyond his understanding. "I'll get right on this, Mrs. Casbah."

"Yes, do!"

She wandered around the store, intent on entertaining herself while Alex collected her groceries that her housekeeper used to cook their meals. Besides, she didn't need some man to sing the praises about some *cripple* who'd come to town and captured the fancy of her son. How could some *cripple* play piano? She'd been to enough concerts with her husband that she knew any piano player had to use their feet for it to sound like anything. No *cripple* could do that! There was no way anything she played could sound like some angel! And to paint like that? No way! Painters didn't use their feet to paint, but still.... There had to be something wrong with a person's brain to be crippled, right?

Millie stood glaring at the back of the little square in the window so long that she jumped when Alex said, "Mrs. Casbah, I have your list finished and rung up. Will you put that on Derek's charge or pay for it today?"

She waved her hand at the store owner. Was the man an imbecile or what? "I didn't bring my purse in, put it on his account. He'll pay up at the end of the month. You know his money's good, good thing you hurried, I got some place to go."

Alex turned away and shook his head, as he found a bag to fill. How could any man put up with a woman like this? No wonder her first husband had run off! He was pretty sure he knew why Ramon went off for days at a time he couldn't stand his mom making a pest out of herself whenever he was in town and he knew she did every chance she could. As he put the last of the bags in the cart ready to push out to her car, he wondered what would ever happen if Ramon got serious about a woman. Millie would probably come to the wedding and tell the preacher she had an objection.

When Alex had all the bags in her car he closed the trunk. Millie hadn't even watched him, but started up and looked at the clock on her dash. Ramon hadn't told her how long he planned to mow or where his plans would take him this afternoon. If she drove by his place again so that she could see if he was still mowing, he'd see her and know she was snooping. How could she follow him when she didn't know how soon he was leaving or where his plans took him? Besides, she remembered seeing some frozen steaks and a tub of ice cream in the things in the trunk, she'd have to go home and unload first. She sighed maybe this wasn't the time to follow her son. But she would! Absolutely! She'd have no part of her perfect son ruining his life over some *cripple*. Angry that her plans had been thwarted, Millie raced the motor then yanked the stick from park jammed her foot on the accelerator, and burning rubber as she pulled away from the little grocery store.

Derek was the bank president of the largest bank in Blairsville. He was a busy man, making all the money he could to keep his unhappy wife as happy as he could. He stayed late at work and arrived early in the mornings, so Saturdays he liked to stay home for a leisure day and do something different. While he read the morning paper, she'd come in the den and informed him she was going for a drive. He'd looked at her, she was dressed fit to kill, but it didn't turn his head as it once had. Now he only wondered what he'd ever seen in her back then. He'd learned over the years that she did that for herself, not for him.

Several hours later, he heard the garage door go up and sighed, soon, his peaceful morning would be shattered. She was always coming up with some bombshell. The woman came in through the kitchen door and said to the housekeeper, "I bought your list of stuff. It's in my car. You'd better go get it, there's ice cream that'll melt and ruin my trunk."

"Yes, Ms. Casbah," the seventy something lady told the forty something lady.

Without so much as a reply, Millie came to the door of the den. "So, you're here!"

"Yes, where did you think I'd be on a Saturday morning, Millie?"

She waved her hand out the window. "It's a nice day, maybe out driving around, who knows, or playing golf with some buddies."

"Millie, I drive back and forth to Blairsville every day, why should I go out for a drive on Saturday when I don't have to?" he asked, reasonably. "Golf; not my style."

She slouched into a chair, letting her tight skirt ride up her thighs intentionally and without becoming upset in any way, she said, "I want a divorce."

Derek looked at her astonished. "What? What for?"

Millie shrugged. "I want out!"

"How would you support yourself? Where would you live?"

"Alimony. I'd live here."

Derek shook his head. "No, Millie. We signed a prenuptial agreement, as you insisted, I might add. There'd be no alimony and this house was mine before I married you, it was never redeemed. Millie, would you be interested to know that you'd have nothing? You haven't worked a day since you married me, but you spend everything you had and the credit cards I've given you are maxed out every month. No, you'd be in really bad shape if you divorced me."

"I… I'd live with Ramon," she said, grasping at straws.

Derek shook his head again. "I don't think so, Millie, Ramon has his own life, his own place. I know for a fact that his mother wouldn't be welcome to live under his roof. He surely wouldn't support you in the way you're used to and besides, suppose someday he finds a young lady to marry. They wouldn't want you living with them." *I guarantee that.* he added silently, *I don't even want to live with you!*

"He won't marry!" she said with a sneer. "He's never home no woman wants her husband gone all the time like he is."

Derek shrugged. Knowing he'd said all he was going to, he picked up the paper again. Peeking around the edge, he said, "You never know. He may quit for her or she might go with him. So is it a divorce or not?"

Pushing from the chair, but making sure her tight skirt stayed mid-thigh on the way, she headed for the hallway. From the doorway, Millie said, "I'll think about it and let you know."

"Fine!" Derek watched her out of sight, then sighed and went back to his paper. He was pretty sure there would be no divorce on her part. She liked the money she had access to too much for such a drastic move. Now him, it wasn't such a bad idea, now that he thought about it. Move her out and move in one of the young things from the bank…. Now that was something to think about! Maybe one of these days….

Ramon nearly ran behind his mower. He set it really high for the first time over he knew he'd never keep it running if he tried to mow it all off the first time around. When he finished mowing the first time, he looked at his watch and sighed, he had fifteen minutes before he should be at Sandy's. He didn't even have to raise his arm to know he must shower first before going.

He pushed the mower into his storage shed and went in the house. It was a warm day, shorts were in order. He wondered if Sandy ever wore shorts. He'd seen her in slacks and a dress, but never shorts. Even last night in her cabin she'd had slacks on. Did her religion tell her she couldn't or was it her choice? He shrugged. She didn't have long hair done up in one of those rats nests, probably there wasn't a dress code, either.

The minute hand was inching toward the twelve as he drove down the street toward the other end of town. He hoped she didn't think he'd stood her up. He sighed; his mom picked the worst times to come. Second only were her phone calls. Usually they lasted longer than her visits. Wasn't Derek keeping her busy? He had a thought that made him shudder. If they ever divorced would she want to live with him? The thought nearly made him loose the granola bar he'd crammed in his mouth only a few minutes ago. He was a grown man surely she wouldn't do that to him! He sighed again she was ornery and cantankerous enough to want to.

Sandy got up early. She listened to the weather as she brushed her teeth and knew it would be a warm day. She sighed, she had one pair of shorts, but her legs looked so anemic and spindly that she didn't want to wear them, especially going with Ramon for the very first time. Who knew where they'd go, if they'd see anyone. Besides, she didn't really know Ramon too well, he'd been gone most of the time since she'd come.

She put on her coolest slacks and a very cool top, brushed her hair and added a hint of lipgloss and put sandals on her feet. She fixed her breakfast then started lunch for them. When Ramon finished up her spaghetti last night, she'd concluded that he didn't eat very well on his own. The lunch she'd make would be a cold dinner. Besides, if he'd mowed all morning he was probably hungry from all that work. At eleven o'clock he wouldn't stop for anything to eat.

She fixed fried chicken then wrapped each piece in paper towels to absorb the grease before she put them in a big baggy. She made a pudding pie with fancy sprinkles on top for dessert, glad that she'd bought some pie crusts at Alex's when she went shopping. She threw in carrot sticks, pickle chips, tomatoes and celery, spread with creamed cheese. She opened a tin of biscuits, put them in the oven and decided she had enough to fill a young man up. Last of all, she made a gallon of iced tea with lots of ice cubes to keep it really cold. She was excited, wondering where he'd take her.

She looked at the clock he should be here any minute! She took her basket and thermos on her lap to the door, then went to her closet and pulled out painting supplies, a canvas and her easel. With scenery like this, if there was a possibility of a picture, she'd be prepared. She also found her camera. If she couldn't paint on this outing, she could take pictures and paint them later, but painting the actual scene was always best. Another look at the clock told her he was running a little late. She wouldn't worry, not yet, he was home so little, there were probably things she couldn't even think of he had to do.

She had just had that thought when she heard a truck drive up out front. A smile captured her lips as she wheeled herself to the door. A handsome young man wearing shorts came around the back of his truck. She sucked in her breath, hiking all those miles didn't do him a bit of harm! His legs looked tanned and solid. Oh, for legs like that!

She waited until he was on the porch to open the door, but she didn't let him knock. As she opened the door, she exclaimed, "Ramon! You look great again! Two times now you haven't been in hiking gear."

He grinned and his eyes twinkled. He basked under her praise. "Thanks. Your place smells terrific. What is it?"

"Probably the fried chicken. I have a few things I'd like to take and since we're taking the van there's plenty of room. I didn't get anything out there yet, though."

He looked at the picnic basket and thermos, then at the pile of everything else. "You think you'll paint?"

Sheepishly, she said, "If it won't bore you, but I brought my camera so I can take pictures and paint from them."

He picked up the basket and thermos, knowing that a camera would work better and they'd get to see a lot more. He wouldn't deny her the opportunity to paint, however. "We have lots of places to see, but we don't have to do them all in one afternoon, I guarantee that. In fact, we can't possibly see them all."

"Ramon, I want to see all I can! Who knows when I'll get out again to see these lovely scenes!" Sandy loaded up her lap and followed him out the door. Because the end of her walk was wide, she was able to reach the locks for the lift from it, so she stuck the key in first one, then the other. As soon as the lift was on the ground, she said, "Why don't you ride the lift and put those things down in the back, then go back for my easel while I get on? Once everything's in, we can close up the van and rearrange the seats to suit us."

"Sure! I've never ridden a lift into a vehicle before. I guess an elevator or escalator's about my limit so far."

She chuckled. "Today's a first for me I never rode on the passenger side before."

When he was back with the easel, Sandy closed the door from the inside, then sat out of the way and said, "The man at the dealership showed me how to take the seat out and there are pictures in the owner's manual in the glove box. You'd probably better get out the pictures, I'm not one to explain things very well that I don't know how to do myself. I think I'll be in the way and not much help, so I'll stay back here."

Standing beside her, with his head bent, Ramon looked at the front of the van. It was weird to see an empty place behind the steering wheel. There was a gas pedal and brake pedal in the usual place on the floor, but there were many gadgets on the dash and steering column that were never on a normal car like his. He went to the seat on the passenger side and sat down, then opened the glove box and found the book. He turned sideways to include her in the instructions, then found the place in the book that said how to convert the van so that a traditional driver could operate it and began to read.

He looked up at Sandy and said, "It says to do a little work over there before setting the driver's seat in position. Guess that's first."

Sandy shrugged. "I guess you'll have to follow directions, my driving instructor always had to crawl down under the steering wheel to fix things."

Ramon chuckled. "I guess that's my job, then."

She gave him one of her fantastic smiles and said, "I guess you're right." She chuckled. "The van's so new I haven't had a chance to get it dirty."

Since neither of them had done it before, it took about twenty minutes to get the seat moved and the van ready for Ramon to drive. When the seat was behind the wheel, Sandy anchored her chair in the grooves where the seat had been and Ramon moved behind the wheel. He'd never driven a new vehicle before, so he appreciated the engine's purr when he started up.

"This is a nice van, Sandy."

"Thanks." She made a face and added, "Unfortunately, I had to wait until I had saved enough money to buy a new one with all these bells and whistles. My brother bought his first clunker last year and he's two years younger than me."

Ramon chuckled. "Yeah, I had one of those, too."

He drove down the street, going by his house then left the little town. Sandy sighed as she looked out the window. "Ramon, you can't know how much I love the out-of-doors!"

He'd only been gone from Isabel's cabins for about ten minutes when a Jaguar drove onto the gravel. Isabel sighed, knowing who the driver was, but she didn't move from her desk. If Millie Casbah wanted to see her for anything she must come inside. She'd seen Ramon and Sandy working inside the van, but she hadn't come out to be nosy. She was happy for Ramon, finally showing some interest in a young lady. Sandy couldn't be a bad choice. She knew Ramon had no religious beliefs, but if anyone could stir anything in him, Sandy could, for sure.

Isabel watched the Jaguar. For several minutes Millie only sat in it. She had to see that Ramon's truck was there, but the blue van was not. She wondered what Millie thought of her son going on a date with someone who was handicapped. Finally the woman left the car and came purposefully toward her office. Isabel nearly laughed out loud, she looked ridiculous. She could hardly walk in those shoes on her gravel parking lot. Her grin nearly split her face as she watched the woman, but before Millie barged through her door, she made her face as bland as possible. Millie Casbah wasn't one to laugh at herself.

Millie barged through the door without knocking. Without saying any greeting, Millie spat out the words, "Is my son here? His truck is."

Feeling ornery, Isabel said, "Well, good afternoon to you, Millie. How are you today? No, Ramon left a little while ago. I didn't ask and he didn't tell me where."

"You should have," she accused, angrily. "I need to know where he went!"

"Why? He's an adult he comes and goes as he pleases. My parking lot has no fence around it I can't keep people in or out."

Acting as if she hadn't heard what Isabel said, Millie said, "Alex at the store told me that *cripple* lives here. Did he go with her?"

Isabel saw red. She jumped from her chair and leaned over so that she was almost in Millie's face. "Listen here, Mildred Casbah, that's the last time you call Sandy such a disgraceful name! She's a wonderful young woman, one doesn't notice the chair."

Millie stepped back from Isabel, unfazed by Isabel's outburst. "Is he out with her?"

"Does it matter?"

"Of course! No son of *mine* goes out with a woman only half there!" she exclaimed. "I demand you tell me where he is!"

Isabel had had enough of this arrogant woman. She had never liked the woman, even when she was unmarried and had her little son and moved to town. She walked around her desk, took the woman firmly by the arm and without a word, ushered her to the door. Millie was so surprised she didn't give any resistance. In fact, she couldn't her shoes tangled up as Isabel turned her. Still holding her firmly, Isabel opened the door and pushed her out, then as Millie staggered from the slight change from inside, across the threshold to the porch, she said, "That's the last time you speak down about one of my renters. You're not welcome on my property again, Millie Casbah. You're the world's worst! I can't understand what your husband sees in you at all! Thank goodness your son didn't turn out like you! Get off my property and don't ever come back here!"

Finally, before she toppled off the porch, Millie found her footing and stomped down the steps to the gravel lot. She took one step in the gravel and her shoes made her ankle twist so that she went down. Isabel still stood at the door, but rather than feel sorry for Millie, she turned and closed the door between them. She stepped back, but watched as the woman pushed herself up and dusted herself off. She tried for another step, but nearly went down again. She righted herself and looked back at the office and made a face at it, but didn't see Isabel watching her, which was just as well. Isabel wasn't sure what either of them would do if she had.

She limped to her car, but Isabel muttered, "Serves her right! I wish… well, no, I can't wish something like that on her it wouldn't do the Lord any service. But sometimes I wish that woman didn't live in this town!"

Ramon drove out into the hills that he hiked in day after day, spring through fall, but of course, he kept to the roads. The day was beautiful, only wisps of white clouds in a deep blue sky. They were comfortable in the air conditioned van. Sandy's head was going back and forth every minute trying to take in everything. The smile that everyone knew her by was firmly on her lips and her eyes were sparkling. Her hands moved constantly, Ramon was enchanted watching her as she enjoyed the countryside. He loved these hills and hollows, but he realized he was gaining a new appreciation of his world as he saw it for the first time through her eyes. One thing for sure, he was eternally grateful for the use of his legs.

After several minutes of just looking out the window, Sandy clapped her hands and grinned at him. She exclaimed, "Ramon, this is wonderful! Thank you for bringing me! You can't know how I love getting out in God's beautiful world. There's a park not too far from my parents' home where I've gone to paint, but I think I've painted every inch of the place and I was so tired of it. This is all new and so much better. There are mountains, or hills, whatever you call them that aren't back there at all. You know, I think I could find my own way out here some time to paint."

"Yes, you probably could. Up the road a little ways is a gravel road that leads to a place I thought we'd stop for our lunch. Are you hungry?"

Sandy laughed. "I can eat, but I've heard your stomach growl a time or two. Tell me if I'm nosy, but did you eat breakfast?"

Ramon chuckled. "You caught me. I overslept and didn't wake up until I heard knocking at the door. It was my mom and she wasted over half an hour of my mowing time. I had a cup of coffee and a granola bar."

Her eyes still twinkling, she slammed her fists on the armrests of her chair and exclaimed, "Ramon DeLord, you get to this place pronto! I had a feeling you don't eat right when you're home by yourself. This proves I'm right. I'm glad I made a real meal rather than throwing some sandwiches together."

Taking one hand from the wheel, Ramon pointed and said, "The pull off's right up here, we'll be there in a second."

As they went around the curve, Sandy said, "Your mom came over. Does she always dress like she's meeting the Queen of England?"

Without hesitation, Ramon said, "Yes. At first I think it was to impress her new husband, but now I think it's to make herself presentable in her own eyes."

"I hate to say this, but she wasn't very nice when she came over that day."

"Sandy, she's not nice. There's a word I won't say in your presence that fits her to a tea."

"Oh, Ramon, your own mother?"

"Yes, my own mother! I don't see how her husband can stand her, except that he spends long hours at his bank in Blairsville. He and I don't like each other much, but I feel sorry for him being strapped with that woman. Of course, that keeps her away from me some. She really gets bent out of shape if she knows I've been home and don't call her while I'm home. She came by in her Jag this morning, but then wanted me to take her to Blairsville to the mall."

"In her car or yours?"

"I don't know. I didn't care enough to ask."

He pulled up into a small picnic area with a breathtaking view before them. "Here we are, Sandy. Two feasts here, one for the stomach and one for the eyes."

Sandy looked out the windshield and gasped. "Ramon! This is so awesome! God makes everything beautiful! Thank you for this."

She wasted no time, but unhooked the locks that kept her chair in place and backed out of the spot. Ramon stood crouched over, his head brushing the ceiling of the van, waiting for her. "Do you want to get your easel out?"

"No, I've decided I can paint these scenes another day. I want to spend the time with you and let you show me everything there is to see. There's so much around every curve and if I stop to paint, what would you do?"

"Okay, it's the basket and thermos then?"

"Yes. We can use one of those tables, can't we?"

"Sure."

"I'll put my camera around my neck."

When they were on the ground, Sandy wheeled herself to one of the tables with a full view of the awesome scenery. She went to an end and Ramon placed the basket and thermos in front of her. Sandy opened the basket, pulled out a bright tablecloth then gave the basket and thermos back to Ramon. She flicked out the cloth and it fell nicely over their end of the table. Ramon set the basket down in front of her again then sat beside her. She pulled out plates, silverware and plastic glasses, then pulled out bags of food, enough for an army, Ramon thought.

With his second piece of chicken in his hands, Ramon asked, "I hope you don't mind my asking, but how did you become handicapped?"

Looking off toward the faraway hills, she took a deep breath. Even though the view was awesome, Ramon knew she wasn't looking at it as she said, "It happened a long time ago in the hospital nursery." Ramon nearly choked on the piece of chicken he was trying to swallow. "I have never walked because on my second day of life the nurse who was changing me dropped me against the side of the changing table. I try not to think about it and I rarely tell people about it. If I dwell on it I could become a bitter woman. My dad encouraged me for as long as I can remember to do as much as I could with what I had. My brother and sister have never let me get away with anything. I'm glad for them and their support, without it, I'd probably be working some no-count job in a place especially for handicapped people. I love my mom, but she's the exact opposite. She has always tried to keep me back."

Ramon shook his head. "You are amazing, Sandy. Several times I've forgotten that you're even in that chair. Your love of life and your attitude make me forget."

She smiled it reached even beyond to her eyes and covered him. "I'm glad, Ramon, that's been my goal all my life. I don't want people to feel sorry for me I want them to think of me as a normal person as much as possible. Sure, there are always those who don't and I know that, but I'm glad for people like you who do."

"You honor me, Sandy," Ramon said, sincerely.

Sandy shook her head. "No, Ramon, you honor me."

It was Saturday. Charlie and Ed both had the day off. Charlie could never sleep in his inner alarm always woke him at the same time no matter what day of the week it was. Colleen slept as Charlie quietly pulled on some scruffy clothes and headed for his workbench downstairs. He knew he had at least an hour before any interruptions came and he loved to work in the early morning. Sandy had always been up shortly after him and she had done much of the painting for him, but now he had to do it himself. He sighed, but he wouldn't wish her back. Just as he thought, about an hour later, he heard Colleen bustling around in the kitchen over his head. He hadn't heard her get up, the basement didn't extend to the very front of their house, but he heard her humming to herself. That was a good sign, she hadn't done that much since Sandy left.

About fifteen minute later, he heard, "Charlie, Ed, breakfast's ready!"

Charlie finished what he was doing then headed for the stairs. He and Ed walked into the kitchen at about the same time, but Charlie went to the sink and washed his hands. Colleen had pancakes on a plate, bacon and eggs on another. The kitchen smelled wonderful. There were tall glasses of orange juice at each place and coffee steaming in the mugs. The cream and sugar sat in front of Ed, he was the only one who doctored his coffee. Charlie couldn't tolerate doctored coffee, you drank it strong and black in the old country.

After Charlie said grace, Colleen waited until both men had a mouthful before she asked, "How long does it take to get to north Georgia?"

Charlie swallowed first and said, "I don't know, Mama. It'd take several hours to leave the city, I'd suspect. I'm sure it's quite a few hours to drive the rest. The trucking company said they'd get Sandy's piano to her Tuesday afternoon. They had their truck nearly full, so Ed says, when they came. Not knowing where we're going, it'd take us a good while, I'm sure. Why?"

Looking between them, but not at either of them, she said, "I have a bad feeling about Sandy. We need to go get her and bring her home."

"What kind of bad feeling, Mama?"

"It's that man she's working for. We need to get her away from him." She wouldn't look at either of the men at the table. In fact, she looked at her plate and studiously worked on the pancake on her plate.

"Mom?" Ed said, setting his fork down on his plate and waited for her to look at him. "Has she called to say she needs rescuing?"

Her eyes fell immediately, she wouldn't look at him. She picked up the knife to spread butter on her pancake. "Of course not! She'd never admit she can't handle things, but I know, here in my mother's heart. She needs to be home." She put her knife down and patted her chest.

Charlie put his hand over her other one as it lay on the table. After a minute, while she looked at his hand on hers, he said, "Mama, Sandy has her own vehicle. She is twenty-five years old. Unless we hear from a hospital in that area saying that we need to come because our daughter is sick or injured, we will not be going down there until we're invited."

Colleen yanked her hand from underneath Charlie's and put it on the chair arm. With fire in her eyes, she yelled, "You're not her mother you don't know what I know!"

Ed slugged down half his glassful of juice, then said, "Tell us, Mom. I'm anxious to know what you know without word from anyone."

Colleen glared at her son. "Edwin, be respectful of your mom! I know in my heart, it's a mother thing. No father or brother can possibly know!"

Shaking his head, Ed said, "Mom, I'm not disrespectful, not at all. I'm telling you like it is. Dad's right, unless you're invited or some hospital down there calls, you need to leave her alone. Besides, how would you get everything home? You'd have to hire the trucking company again to bring back her piano and they'd think you were off your rocker! Besides, you can't drive her van, it's handicapped equipped. Besides, how do you know there's anything wrong with the man who hired her?"

Instantly, she stuck her nose in the air and answered, "I wouldn't have let it go in the first place! I don't care now if it comes back. She'd have her painting. Of course, that is if she's in any condition to do anything when she gets back!" Colleen said dramatically. "You have no idea, you or your dad!"

Turning to his dad, Ed asked, "Did Sandy give you a phone number?"

"Yes, we got a letter the other day. She sent an address and phone number."

"Maybe you ought to call before anyone makes a foolish decision about going down those hundreds of miles for nothing."

"Edwin, it's not for nothing!" Colleen cried. "I know what I'm feeling, she needs to come home! And… and it needs to be really soon!"

"Mom, *you're* feeling she needs to come home. The real question is, does she?"

"Of course she does!" she whispered. "Besides, if you call, she'll say there's no need and that man'll do something even worse!"

"Mom?" he again waited for her to look at him. He was beyond getting angry with his mom. "I don't think so. I think you're who's lonely you're trying to put something on Sandy that really is you. You miss her, so you want her back. Dad, could you get away for a few days to take Mom to the country to see Grandma?"

Charlie thought a minute. "I think I could take Monday off. Yes, sure! I could make a few phone calls and we could leave today for a few days. That's a good idea, Son. Yes, it's a good time of year to get out of the city."

Colleen grabbed the arms of her chair and held them tightly, as if someone was going to take her forcefully from the table to the car and take her somewhere she didn't want to go. North instead of south. "No! We will go to Georgia and bring Sandy home!"

Just as vehemently, Charlie shook his head. "No, Mama, we won't. Unless she calls or someone calls with some news, we will not go to Georgia!"

EIGHT

Still holding the armrests in a death grip, Colleen cried, "You just don't understand! You don't know a mother's heart." She was nearly hysterical.

Trying valiantly to hide his pity, Charlie said, "Yes, Colleen, you're right, I don't understand and I don't have a mother's heart, but I do have a father's heart and I know that for many years you've tried your best to keep Sandy from being all that she can be. She's living as close to her potential as she can, but no thanks to you."

Colleen could only gasp. She swallowed and gasped again. "How can you say that?"

"Dad can say that because it's absolutely true, Mom." Ed stood up and took his plate to the sink. "Give it up, Mom. It's not your place to go rescue her." He looked out the window and made a face. "I think I'd better mow the grass, it's the pits."

After Ed left and the mower started, Colleen said, "Charlie, we must go for Sandy!"

"Why? She didn't call this morning, did she?"

"No. She's in trouble, though."

"You have vision that sees over the miles?"

"Don't make fun of me, Charles!"

"I'm not Colleen. I think it's really sad what you're putting yourself through because Sandy's gone away against your wishes.

As I've already said several times, we're not going to north Georgia until we're invited. She said she'd probably be home for Christmas. If that's not soon enough for you, I'm sorry." He smiled at his wife almost sure what her reaction would be to what he would say next. "Besides, maybe she'll call and invite us down for her wedding!"

Colleen slapped her hands back on the arms of her chair and reared out of the seat. "Charles! How can you say that? She's not getting married!"

"No, not right now, but she might."

Charlie had never seen his wife get so upset in such a short time. Her eyes glistened, but she didn't cry. Hysterically, she said, "She's not getting married! She can play for a wedding, she can sing at a wedding, but she's never getting married!"

He looked at his wife and asked, calmly, "And you know this because?"

She sank back in the chair, tears sliding down her cheeks. "She's a *cripple*! No man wants a cripple for a wife!"

Charlie was out of his chair and around the table almost before Colleen knew what had happened. "Colleen," he picked her up by her upper arms and looked her square in the eyes. "Colleen, there may be a very special man out there who will love her regardless of her **handicap** and want only her to be his wife. Don't, absolutely **do not** put yourself in God's place and say she will never get married!" Colleen gasped, but had nothing to say.

Ramon eyed the last two pieces of chicken still in the bag. He sighed and saw the pie Sandy had pulled from the picnic basket. He rubbed his full stomach, stifled a burp and shook his head. How could this woman cook so well? His mom had never been a cook, they'd eaten frozen dinners for as long as he could remember and they were still his main food source. He didn't think Sandy knew what a frozen dinner was.

Wiping his mouth on his napkin, he said, "Sandy, you have outdone yourself two meals in a row! This is terrific! I'm about full enough to pop and still you have more."

Sandy shrugged, accepting his praise without comment and said, "I see a pretty wide trail over there, could we take it for a bit, then come back for some pie?"

"Sure! Where's your camera, can I get it for you?"

"Would you? It's there on the back seat. I forgot to pick it up even after I said I would."

Ramon went to the passenger door and opened it. It was a weird feeling to step up two steps and not have to sit down in the seat, but keep on walking to the back of the van to the back seat. He found the camera easily, it wasn't some little disposable job you buy at a department store it was one of those you must focus for each picture. If she made a painting from one of her pictures, it would be first quality.

He hurried back with it and she reached for it. "Here, the strap is the right length that it sits in my lap so it won't bounce or get in the way. Lead on, oh fearless one, lead on!" She smiled and put out her hand toward the trail.

Ramon took a step and he heard the motor on Sandy's chair start. That was the first time he realized what it was. When they reached the trail, he said, "Sandy, it's wide enough and easy to follow, I'll walk beside you so we can talk."

"Thank you. You're so considerate, Ramon, I appreciate that."

Most of the walk Sandy was exclaiming about the awesome views. She made Ramon stop several times so she could take pictures. She was very precise with her settings and her lens. He realized she could probably sell her photos if she wanted. He wondered what she'd say about the pictures he'd taken with his little camera that were now at the shop being developed. He loved taking pictures and knew he did a fair job, but he'd never had a camera like hers.

About half an hour later they came to the end of the trail. There was a metal barricade across the end and in front of them was wide open space that let them see for miles and miles across a valley with trees and a river far below. He heard her gasp, but she said nothing as her head went back and forth taking in every angle, every rise and fall in the terrain. Without taking her eyes from the view, she pulled her camera from its case and brought it to her eyes. After focusing, she snapped two pictures, but then they both heard the camera start to rewind.

She sighed, as she lowered the camera, letting the camera do its thing. "Ramon, where can I get my film printed and buy more film?"

"Brad Thomas, at the gas station has a photo section where you can take your film and buy more. He doesn't have a one hour option, since he doesn't do it, but the pictures are usually back within a week."

The film finished winding, so she took it out, dropped it in the case then pulled out a fresh roll. "That's okay. I talked to him about putting up a sign for me. He seems nice."

Dubiously, Ramon looked at her. "Are we both talking about the Brad Thomas who runs the gas station/hardware store?"

Sandy shrugged a twinkle in her eyes. "I bought gas there and asked if he'd put up my ad for piano lessons. He took my gas money and put my sign in the window."

Ramon shook his head, a half smile on his face. "Sandy, that man has rare days when he's civil. Most of the time he's a grouch. Believe me, I've lived in this town for over ten years and I've never known the man to be nice."

She grinned at him, her eyes twinkling and said, "After he put the sign in the window, he asked how I taught piano and I moved my fingers in front of me and said, 'Oh, beginners move their ten fingers up and down the keys.' He smiled and said, 'Well, perhaps I meant how do *you* play piano?' Before I could answer he said, 'I know you move your ten fingers up and down the keys, but don't you have to use your feet?' I assured him that most pianists did, but I had a piano that knew what it was supposed to do without me using mine."

Ramon threw his head back and laughed. Hiccoughing, he exclaimed, "Oh, Sandy! You are something else. I bet you made his day."

She shrugged. "Perhaps I did, I didn't stay to find out. I was in a hurry you know and had to get back to get that first call."

She loaded the new roll of film into her camera and finished taking the rest of the panorama before her. After putting her camera back into its case, she looked up at him and said, "I guess we go back and keep on?"

"Yes, but I'd like to show you something first."

"Oh, sure!"

Pointing to their right, he said, "See that stand of trees over there?" When she nodded, he said, "I bring my groups to that point and camp there the last night we're out. There's a nice stream there that's mountain fed. People like to drink the water, it tastes fresh and pure every time we stop there and it's so cold even on a hot day it feels like it comes from the refrigerator."

"That'd be great to drink, but not too nice to swim in."

"Yeah, that's true, but some do." She shivered at that.

Loving how she responded to his explanations, he turned toward the west and pointed again. "On Labor Day, when I take that group of seasoned hikers and Duncan Roads we'll drive down the road a little farther from where we're parked, then go off on a dirt trail. We'll hike in those woods and hills for our three days."

"It looks sort of wild over there. What kind of wildlife do you have?"

"There are some bears in the Appalachians Once in a while we hear a big cat in the evening, but mostly it's coyotes or foxes. Perhaps we'll find a snake across the path, but there are lots of rabbits, squirrels and deer roaming around, maybe a skunk."

"I don't want you to put yourself into any danger, but if you can get a good shot at one of those bigger beasts I'd love to paint from the picture."

He nodded. Thinking about his own little box, he said, "I'll see what I can do. Of course, my camera isn't as sophisticated as yours is."

Shaking her head, she said, "Ramon, I lived at home for twenty-five years. My parents never took money for room and board from me. I've taught piano for well over six years, getting an income from it. I've sold my paintings since I was a young teenager and had a gallery for my paintings for several years. My dad's hobby is making things in his workshop and I've painted them for him. When he sells them, he's given me a percentage of his profit. What have I had to spend my money on except a fancy camera and a handicapped equipped van and some clothes? Nothing. I rarely go anywhere but to church. You on the other hand, have lots of expenses."

His admiration growing exponentially, he said, "I'll be glad to take some pictures. Don't be disappointed, though if I don't get any wild animals, they're pretty shy with a group of hikers. Two trips ago we stopped at a really beautiful place for the night. The sunset was awesome and made the lighting spectacular for pictures, so I took some with you in mind. That roll of film is at the developers right now. I'll let you have them when they come back."

"Super! I'll be anxious to see them."

He leaned against the metal railing, his back to the view, but he could look at her. He loved to see her expressions, not only the ever-present smile and said, "This last group of three couples was impressed with my painting. One girl wanted to come next week and ask if you'd paint her a picture. Another girl, who was half of the newlywed couple that went, was interested when I told them you'd painted a portrait for your landlady." He grinned. "She looked up at her husband and batted her eyelashes at him and insisted they must have you paint their portrait."

Sandy laughed. "I'll agree to both if they come back."

"No one will ever get my painting," he said, fiercely, "but if you want to paint some and have me hang them to sell, I'll be glad to do that."

"Thanks, I know you said that, but I've been doing some things around my cabin and getting caught up on my piano playing this week. In the afternoons next week, I'll probably come back out here and start some canvasses. I'll have you some soon." She sighed and looked out at the panorama again. "This is so awesome! God made a beautiful world for us to live in."

Ramon pushed away from the railing and took her hand, then took a step, so Sandy moved her control to turn around. "I don't know, Sandy, maybe He did."

It was nearly dusk when they returned to Sandy's cabin. Ramon pulled up to Sandy's spot and shut off the van. Sandy backed out of the way and Ramon started the job of reversing the seats and putting the driving mechanism back to hand controls. It didn't take quite as long to put it back. Ramon found it really wasn't hard, once he knew what he was doing.

Isabel waited until the lift came down, then she went out and walked over to them. "Your mom was here just after you left, Ramon."

He groaned. "What did she want, Isabel?"

She shook her head and snorted. "To know where you'd gone and not very nicely asked if Sandy had gone."

Ramon made a face. "I hope you didn't tell her anything! I can imagine what she said."

Isabel scowled and said fiercely, "I told her never to come back to my property again! I would not tolerate her saying things like she said about my renters again."

Sandy wheeled herself over to Isabel and hugged her. "Isabel, you are priceless! Thanks for defending me. I've had a run-in with her already, she wasn't very nice."

"She's not!" She looked at Ramon, but then said, "If I had my way, she'd be run out of town on a rail, not just off my property!"

Ramon nodded and said, sincerely, "I'm with you, Isabel. Ever since everything's been given to her by her husband, she's become intolerable." He looked down at Sandy and said, "Can I take these things in for you?"

Sandy shrugged. "I'd be glad for you to carry the easel in. You must take the basket home and finish up what's there. I'll get it next week. What time do you leave tomorrow?"

"I guess this is another church group. They asked if they could come and start about two. By then it's almost silly to start out, four hours is about all you can go before we must set up camp so it's not too dark to fix supper."

She smiled at him, knowing his response. "Great, you could go to church with us!"

He heard Isabel chuckle, knowing that Isabel went to church, but he ignored her and said, "Sandy, you know I don't do church! I never have as an adult perhaps I did as a wee child. This is the first summer I've had groups who've said 'grace' over their meals. That's a new concept for me. I know you're into this God thing, but I'm not."

She smiled and patted his hand. "I know we'll work on that, though. He's the best thing that could happen to anyone, you'll see."

With her easel in his hands, he asked, "You know that?"

"Yes! Some time when we have more time I'll explain it to you more. You said you have some things to get ready for tomorrow, so it can't be tonight."

"All right, I'll hold you to that." Ramon said, as Isabel turned and went to her place.

Inside her cabin, Sandy wheeled herself in the closet and put her painting things away. Over her shoulder, she said, "That easel goes in here, Ramon. Thanks for bringing it in." As he walked in behind her, she said, "I had the most fantastic day! I'm refreshed and inspired from all the beauty I saw. You'll never know how much this afternoon did for me. Thanks, so much!"

Stepping in the closet behind her, he said, "It's been my pleasure, believe me, Sandy. I'll be back on Thursday afternoon, but not before you leave and I have a two day outing starting on Friday, so it may be a while before we see each other again. Believe me, I've enjoyed your company and the food you've fixed has been out of this world!"

They were still in the huge closet. She was pulled in and he was behind her. She couldn't turn around until he left, then she'd back out, but he wanted with all his heart to kiss her. He'd expressed in words how he felt, but they didn't say what was truly on his heart. A kiss would be the only way, with his arms around her. Did she ever sit on her couch? Her hair was lovely, but kissing it wouldn't do anything for him. He stifled a sigh and left the small space.

She was aware of him leaving the space behind her, so she put her chair control in reverse and moved from the closet then turned around. She looked up at him and for an instant she read something in his eyes that she'd never seen in anyone's eyes before. His eyes were dark, as he looked at her, but she didn't know how to take the message, she smiled, but it didn't reach her eyes. "Thanks," she whispered, "I had a terrific time, Ramon. The views were awesome." She wheeled herself toward the door and waited for him to follow.

As soon as he saw her reaction, he masked his expression and swallowed his desire with some difficulty. Instead of kissing her on his way to the door, he patted her shoulder and said, "It was a pleasure, Sandy. I'll see you sometime. Like I say, it may not be for over a week, but duty calls."

She watched him pick up the basket from the walk outside her van and go to his truck. As he started up, he tried to make sense of her reaction to his obvious desire. He'd read confusion on her face. It was the first time he'd noticed her smile didn't reach her eyes. He scowled, could a twenty-five year old Sandy Bernard never have a man be interested in her as more than a friend and she didn't know how to respond? He shook his head; that made no sense! Surely she had male acquaintances beside her brother, didn't any of them find her desirable? He couldn't imagine that! He remembered what she'd told him about her family, but surely she knew some men?

He drove home, picked up the basket from the passenger seat and went in his empty house. It wasn't near as welcoming or friendly as a little cabin on the other edge of town. There was a blinking light on his answering machine. She wouldn't be back until Monday to retrieve messages he sighed and hit the button to retrieve the message.

"Call you mom," the disagreeable voice said.

"Sure, Mom, I'd love to talk to you after I've spent the most fantastic afternoon of my life with the most perfectly lovely lady in all the world!" he grumbled and deleted the message.

He took the picnic basket to the kitchen and opened it up. The heavenly smell of fried chicken wafted out and he pulled in a deep breath. Instantly, he determined that not one thing from the basket would find its way into his refrigerator. He made good on his silent promise by pulling out the bag with the fried chicken in it and pulling a plate from his cupboard. Dumping the two pieces on the plate, he pulled out the last two biscuits and the rest of the vegetables and emptied those bags onto the plate. With the plate in one hand, he took the pie from the bottom and went to the table. He snagged a carrot on his way back to the refrigerator for the butter and a can of soda then pulled a knife and fork from his drainer. He sat down to eat and the phone rang. He ignored it, letting the machine pick up.

He could hear the voice clearly down the hall from his office. "Answer the phone, Ramon! We have to talk now!"

He heard the click and mumbled around a mouthful, "No, we don't, Mom."

After dark, the phone rang again and again; Ramon let the machine pick up. Finally, after several more times, she said, "Ramon, I know you're home now. Answer!"

He picked up before the click and said, angrily, "What do you want?"

"Respect!"

"Why?"

"Because you owe me!"

Ramon swallowed, what he really wanted to say he couldn't to his mom. "Why, because you're keeping tabs on every move I make? I don't appreciate your tactics, Mom. I know you went to Isabel's and made a donkey out of yourself."

"What! I did not!"

"She threw you off her property, didn't she?"

"She didn't mean it!" she said, snidely.

"That's not the way I heard it straight from her mouth."

"You can't go out with that woman!"

"You know I went out with what woman?"

"You went out with that *cripple*! I won't have it!"

Clenching his fist at his side, he hissed, "Listen to me, Mrs. Casbah, I will not tolerate you calling Sandy a cripple ever again. I believe Isabel, and the same goes for me. You're not welcome on my property again. Do I make myself clear?" He slammed down the phone and quickly went to the bathroom to shower.

"That woman!" he growled. "Why does she have to be my mother?"

He hadn't heard the phone ring, but when he left the bathroom, she was talking on the answering machine. "...and furthermore, you can't keep me away! I'm your mom I have a right to talk to my only son!"

He picked up the receiver, then without bringing it to his ear, set it back in the cradle. As soon as he was sure she had been disconnected, he lifted the receiver again and placed it beside the cradle. He didn't have to talk to her or listen to her tonight. All the wonderful feelings he'd had when he walked in the door had totally vanished once he'd heard her voice. Later on, he crawled into bed and pulled the covers up under his chin. He turned over and looked out the window, wishing for a repeat of last night when he'd dreamed about one lovely young lady. Now all that came to mind was a despicable, selfish woman.

After Ramon pulled away and was out of sight, Sandy poured the last of the iced tea from the thermos over a glassful of ice. She went to her kitchen table and sat drinking her tea slowly. She'd eaten quite a bit for lunch and since she didn't get much exercise, she knew she didn't need to eat much of anything for supper. What she did need to do was try to figure out what that expression on Ramon's face meant. Her dealings with men were quite limited, but she'd seen what she'd assumed was respect, pity, admiration, friendship and love from her family. She pulled up any experience she'd had with other men, but she couldn't ever remember seeing what Ramon's face had told her. She scowled, she had no idea. What had he been thinking as he looked at her outside her closet? She was sure they were friends, was that a look of friendship? Maybe, since she didn't have many male friends, that was a man's 'friendship' look.

She shrugged it wasn't something she'd figure out tonight. She went to her closet and pulled out her easel, her oils and a canvas. She'd have to send away for more canvasses soon. If she wanted to do all the paintings she had in mind, she'd run out in no time at all. It was nice of Ramon to offer to hang her paintings in his office so she could have some exposure here. She pulled out her tubes of paints and smeared a dollop of her colors on her pallet, then from memory, began to paint the awesome scene she'd looked at the whole time they ate their lunch. It was well past the time when she normally went to bed, but she had finished the painting and it was standing beside the climate control that was cooling her cabin and would dry her picture.

In the morning, she had to hurry, because Isabel would be ready to leave for Sunday school by eight fifteen and she wanted to be ready then, too. She dressed in some cool Sunday clothes, had her Bible on her lap and her keys in her hand when she looked out the front window and saw Isabel come out her door and head toward her van.

She wheeled herself onto the porch and called, "Hi, Isabel! It's beautiful this morning!"

Smiling, the old lady said, "It's one of the best days the Lord has made!"

"I agree."

Sandy was quiet as she drove. She hadn't made sense of Ramon's expression all evening and no inspiration had come to her overnight. She rarely remembered any dreams. She wouldn't see him before he left and probably not again until next week. She enjoyed the trip to church, but still came up with nothing.

She sighed, as she followed another car onto the church parking lot. "I was really serious when I asked Ramon to come to church."

Isabel smiled at the serious young woman. "I know you were, Missy, but give him time. I doubt he's ever been in a church his mama never took him, that I know. She's too self-centered to think of anyone but number one since I've known her. She moved here soon after her first husband left her and Ramon was only small. He likes you, you know."

Sandy smiled at Isabel and said, "I like him. He's been more than fair, renting your cabin and buying my first painting."

When Sandy had engaged the parking brake and turned off the key, Isabel reached over and put her hand on Sandy's, as she started to release her chair from the locks. "No, you don't understand what I mean. Sandy, he likes you."

She scowled and looked into Isabel's face. Nodding, she said, "Yes, you said that twice now. I like him, too."

Isabel wondered if she even knew what she meant. "Sandy, look at me." When she did, Isabel asked, "How do you feel about Ramon?"

A bit confused about Isabel's question, Sandy said, "How do I feel about him?" Isabel nodded. "I think he's a wonderful guy. He's shown me respect always, he's fun to be with and he compliments my painting and my piano playing."

Isabel shook her head and pounded her own chest. "That's not it, Sandy, how do you feel down in here about him?"

Confusion spread on Sandy's face and settled in her eyes. Scowling, she asked, "What do you mean, Isabel!"

Taking a deep breath, realizing the girl didn't know about the ways of a man and woman, she let out her breath. Taking a risk, she said, "Sandy, I'm pretty sure he loves you."

Sandy gasped. "How can you say that, Isabel!"

The old lady shrugged. "I was in love once with a man who loved me for fifty-five years. I saw him look at me many times the way Ramon looked at you yesterday."

"But Isabel, we hardly know each other! We only met a little over a week ago and he's been gone most of that time. I don't understand!" Glancing down at the chair she always sat in, she said, "How? How could he love me?"

They were on the parking lot by now. After raising the lift and closing the door, Isabel patted Sandy's hand as they headed for the handicapped entrance to the church. "Missy, I only had to see my husband the very first time to know he was the only man for me. He courted me for only a few months before he asked me to marry him. I accepted immediately and we were married before a year was over. Now-a-days, men and women marry a lot sooner than that. Maybe that's good and maybe it's not so good, I don't know. But I'll stake my last penny on it that Ramon loves you. Do you love him?"

"I don't know, Isabel." Sandy murmured. "I can't remember a man paying attention to me other than Dad and Ed. Most men sort of look the other way when they see this chair."

"It's to their shame!" she exclaimed.

"Perhaps," she sighed.

They went in and each went to a class. Sandy had been introduced to the college and career class of young adults last week and Isabel, of course went to her ladies class. To make sure all the classes were out on time for church, a bell rang twenty minutes before church started and the adult classes met in the big fellowship hall for a closing song. Isabel got there first, but no one was playing the piano. She scowled and looked around for the lady who usually played.

One of the men teachers, also the superintendent, almost went by her looking hassled. She put out her hand and stopped him. Then she asked, "Where's Monica this morning?"

"She's ill and I didn't know it until now. I'm trying to find our organist to fill in, but I guess she's already in the sanctuary."

"You want someone to play?"

"Yes! Do you know someone who can?"

"Sure I do! You remember Sandy Bernard I introduced last week? She's good!"

The man scowled. "Wasn't she the lady in a wheelchair?" He didn't have to say anything out loud his thoughts were written on his face.

Silently, wondering why so many men were prejudice against people with handicaps, she said, "Yes, she was! You remember, ask her."

Absently, the man nodded. Just then, Isabel saw Sandy wheel herself around the corner. "There she is, ask her!"

The man's face turned cherry red. Sandy saw Isabel and smiled, wheeling herself toward her. The man still stood close to Isabel, but he stuck his finger down between his neck and his collar. When Sandy reached them, he stammered, "Umm, Isabel says I should ask you if you'll play our closing song. I wouldn't ask, but our regular player is ill and I didn't know about it until just now, so I couldn't make other arrangements."

Sandy smiled. "Sure, I'll play, it'll be a pleasure."

"You will?" the man gasped. "Come this way!"

At the piano, he gave her the book and said, "Is there one you know and want to play?" *Isabel thinks this woman in a wheelchair can play?* He didn't say the words out loud, but anyone looking at him could see the question on his face.

Sandy shrugged and said, "Whatever anyone wants."

"How about number one hundred?"

Sandy opened to the page, smiled and began playing softly as the people filed in. The man's eyes turned to saucers, as he stepped back. Isabel sat close by, her smile as broad as the sun. People who were talking stopped and a hush fell over the room. The other classes filed in the room quietly, as they realized what was happening. Sandy was far better than Monica.

When every seat was full, the man cleared his throat and said, "Monica is ill and I didn't know it until now, so Ms Bernard consented to fill in. Let's turn to page one hundred and close with the first and last verses."

When they finished singing, Isabel hurried to Sandy's side. "You don't need that little black pouch to play like an angel!" she whispered.

"It's one thing to play something simple like a hymn it's another to play that other stuff, Isabel. I can hold down the keys from one chord to the next to play a hymn, but those other pieces have too many notes to do that."

The man came over to her with his hand out. "Ms. Bernard, I'm Jake Newman. Thanks for filling in like that. You play like a pro!"

Before Sandy could answer, Isabel said, "Didn't I tell you she could play, Jake Newman? She is a pro, she's played for years and also teaches piano."

"Wow! Where do you live, Ms. Bernard?"

"I'm Sandy and I live in one of Isabel's cabins in Vansville."

"We're glad to have you! Please come back again."

"I intend to, believe me."

The warm sun was streaming in his window when Ramon woke up. Before he opened his door, he went to the window that looked out on the back yard. He'd had a weird dream that involved his house and backyard and he wanted to be sure it had only been a dream, that overnight no one had done something to his yard. He pushed open the drape and looked out. Everything was as it had been the grass was still in desperate need of a mow. The high stuff was down and drying making the yard look like a hay field, but the stubble that was left desperately needed another go over.

He went back and sat on his bed, but continued to look out the window. His dream really had been weird. If he could remember it right, his backyard had morphed into a bedroom suite and his office had sprouted two garage doors, with a light blue van parked inside. He scowled, where had his office gone?

He showered and dressed, then made his way to the kitchen and started his coffee. He saw Sandy's picnic basket on the counter and put the clean pie pan back in it. He looked up at the clock and made a face. She'd already left for church with Isabel. There was no reason to go over there, he wouldn't see her anyway. What did the woman see in church? As far as he could tell, she didn't need any encouragement from anybody; that came from inside herself.

A little voice said, *That's because she has something inside her that you don't have.*

He shrugged and pulled out some eggs. He'd make himself an omelet. He hadn't had one in a long time and today was as good as any to have one. He drank a cup of coffee while he fixed the eggs, then poured another and sat down in his place. He thought about the young lady he'd spent much of the day with yesterday. Yes, she must have something he didn't have. She'd told him she'd never walked, if that had been his fate, he'd be a bitter man by now. Yet she was the most phenomenal woman he'd ever met!

When he finished his meal, he went to his office and right away saw the red light on the answering machine, then remembered he'd taken the phone off the cradle so his mom would stop calling. He went back to the phone in the living room and put the receiver back on the cradle, then went back to the office. He pushed the button to retrieve the messages, but before any of them played, he hit the delete. He didn't want to hear his mom's voice today.

He went over his list, then packed his backpack and brought it to the office, tied his tent on and looked at the clock. He still had several hours before the group came. He leaned back as far as the chair would go, then rolled it back from the desk far enough to put his feet up on top. He wondered what people got out of going to church. He couldn't remember being inside one. Would it collapse if he went into one? Would something or Someone reach out and zap him as he stepped inside? Why did Sandy and Isabel think it was important to be in church every seven days? Was there something magical about the seventh day? What could be the reason?

He shrugged and went to his truck. When he'd left Sandy's yesterday he noticed his gas gauge registered near 'E'. The church in town was across the street from the gas station. Maybe he'd come up with something if he went and got gas while the people were in church. Of course, maybe not, Isabel said she wouldn't go in that church for anything and Sandy had gone with her from the start. He wondered what made the difference, wasn't a church a church?

Ramon drove down the street and turned onto Main Street, then drove down the block to the gas station. He pulled in, shut off the motor and even before he stepped from the truck, he could hear the loud band playing across the street. He looked over to the church, but didn't see anything. The door and windows were closed. He opened his door and was nearly blasted off the lot with the noise. Maybe that was why his was the only vehicle at the gas pumps. He hurried and filled his tank and rushed inside the store.

Brad was behind the counter and when the door closed, Ramon said, "Is that noise from the church across the street?"

"It sure is! You mean you never been around on Sunday before, Ramon?"

"At my place, but never here."

Brad shook his head. "That goes on for half 'n R, from ten thirty to eleven. Fifteen minutes later there's another bout a noise and everybody rushes out. I can't see as they look a lot different, but I'd think bein' that close to that noise'd set some of 'em women's hair into a fritz."

Ramon shook his head. "I hear that!"

"Say, did I hear right? Does that handicapped woman work for you?"

"Yes, Sandy's my receptionist, why?"

He nodded toward the door. "She asked if I'd put her picture in the winda so she could get some pi-ana students. I don't hear no pi-ana in that ruckus across the street."

"What I've heard her play doesn't sound anything like that. It's not noise it's soothing, but also invigorating. She's a master, believe me!"

"I'd like to hear her sometime."

That reminded Ramon of what he'd told Sandy. He looked at the clock and knew if he spent a little more time here he could talk to Roger about getting her a place to give a concert. Too bad the church was the biggest place to hold a crowd in town. Then he wondered, since the noise he heard didn't come from a piano if the church even had one in it. That would be the pits they didn't have any way to move her piano anywhere. Then he wondered if she could only use her piano for the black pouch she had to have to play.

155

He sighed, so many questions and he was leaving in a few hours and she was in Blairsville. He couldn't ask her any of them before he left.

It was quiet across the street when he walked out of the gas station. He looked at his watch, from what Brad said, he could talk to Roger in about twenty minutes. It wasn't that far, he'd take his purchases home and come back. They'd surely be done by then. His hikers weren't scheduled to arrive until two o'clock.

Twenty-five minutes later, Ramon drove back down the street. Most of the cars were gone, but the church door was open. He parked and hurried up the five steps to the open door. He approached and Roger called, "Ramon! What are you doing here?"

"Came to ask some questions."

"Well, ask away."

Stepping inside the door, but stopping to let his eyes adjust, Ramon said, "I heard some racket when I went to get gas half an hour ago."

"Racket!" Roger exclaimed. "We were having praise and worship."

Ramon shrugged. "Sorry. I had to go inside Brad's store to be able to think."

Roger raised one shoulder. "Well, that's because you're not into church, you don't know anything about that. So what are these questions you have?"

By now, Ramon had walked into the building far enough to see that there was indeed a piano in the front corner of the room. "Do you ever allow anything other than church to happen in this building?"

"Sure, we've had chili dinners here. A rock band came in one time, now I'll never do that again, I had too many complaints from my ladies. We had a bake sale once, too. That was a lot of fun. Why do you ask?"

"Have you heard about my new receptionist?"

"You mean that lady in the wheelchair?"

"Yes, Sandy Bernard. Her job with me will be over at the end of October, I'm sure you know that, but she needs a means of income after that. She's been a piano teacher for several years and would like to do it again, but it's a bit hard for her to recruit. Maybe you've seen her ad in Brad or Alex's window?"

"Those beautiful paintings?"

"Yes, she painted them."

"Wow!" The man scowled. "She's… her legs don't work? How can she play?" He shook his head. "I don't mean any disrespect, you know."

"That's what I want to ask you. I heard her the other evening and she plays like a master. She'd be willing to give a concert for the public. I suggested she should, it might help people get over the problem they have with her not moving her feet, but still being able to play. What do you say about using this place?"

"So she's good?" Roger asked, still skeptical

"I've never heard anyone better! Isabel Isaacson insists she plays like an angel."

Roger shrugged. "I suppose we could set it up sometime."

"How about after Labor Day? She said she could be ready by then."

"Yeah, that'd work. Can you set it up or will you have her call me?"

Ramon sighed, "I'm leaving at two o'clock on a hike and won't be back until Thursday afternoon. If you'd set it up, tell her I talked with you."

Roger looked at his watch. "You could go by her place now, couldn't you? Didn't I hear she lives in Isabel's cabin?"

"Yes, but she goes with Isabel to church in Blairsville."

Roger shrugged, looking at his watch. "She'll be home soon, call her, then I'll call later."

"All right, but no fancy moves you old bachelor!"

Roger's eyes twinkled. "Don't tell me the old hard-to-catch-Ramon has fallen for some lovely young lady?"

Pink crept up his neck as he turned to leave the church. "Well… I'm not sure I'd go that far yet, old man."

Roger caught up to his friend and slapped him on the back. "I won't try my well known charm on the piano player, I promise."

"Thanks, I'll give her a call before I leave."

"You do that and let her know I'll be calling as well. I think a concert in this little burg will be a good thing."

NINE

After church, people came up to Sandy even before she moved from the spot on the outside aisle and congratulated her for playing in Sunday school. Several told her how beautifully she'd played, others shook her hand. Isabel still sat in the pew, because Sandy had told her she didn't like to be in the way of people leaving the sanctuary. When most of the people had left their side, Sandy turned around and headed toward the door. The main entrance had both stairs and a ramp leading from it.

The pastor came up to shake Sandy's hand. "Ms. Bernard, I hear you rescued my Sunday school superintendent this morning! I want to thank you so much for pinch hitting like that."

Sandy smiled. "It was no problem, Pastor. He picked a simple hymn."

"Could I put you on the list as a substitute?"

"I wouldn't mind, although I'd need to bring my gadget for the sustaining pedal. If you could call me, even the same day before I left, I'd be glad to help out."

"That would be terrific! Thanks so much."

She drove home and there sat a familiar truck in the parking lot. "What's he doing here?" Isabel asked. "Did you invite him for dinner?"

Sandy pulled into her place and answered, "No, he said he had things to do before his group came in to leave at two. I didn't ask him."

Isabel got out of the van while Sandy put the lift down. She stood on the sidewalk and Ramon walked up. "Seen you enough the last couple of days, Sonny."

"Isabel, it's good to see you, too."

She chuckled. "What is this, can't you stay away? You know, that truck of yours has been here a real lot this week."

His eyes twinkled, as he grinned at the older lady, but he wasn't about to answer her question. Isabel could think what she wanted. "I need to ask Sandy something." He checked his watch. "My group'll be here soon, though."

Sandy wheeled herself off the lift then closed up the van before wheeling up to the other two. "So, you wanted to ask me something?"

"Yes, I talked with Roger from the church a bit ago. He said he'd be glad to schedule a concert after Labor Day like we talked about. He said he'd talk with you later on today about it."

She grinned at him. "It'd have to be some evening when you're in town because you'd have to be the MC. I don't do that."

"Me?" he almost squeaked.

"Yup, you. I don't care when, as long as it's after Labor Day. You go check your schedule, then call him and tell him when you can be there."

"Great!" he grumbled. "Me and my big mouth!"

She grinned and patted his arm. "That it is! Have fun on your hike!"

"Mmm, sure!"

"Roger, I guess it's you and me who decide when this concert that Sandy puts on comes off," Ramon said, on a sigh, when Roger answered his phone.

With an obvious frown on his face, Roger asked, "Why's that, man? I thought she was the one playing, not you or me. At least it better not be you or me either as far as I know."

"Mmm, thanks a lot. Actually, I think I'm not that good even with a washboard. However, it seems, when I talked with her that her only two stipulations were that it be after Labor Day and that I be the MC, therefore it had to clear my calendar."

Roger chuckled. "Ahh, I see. So you were the one to suggest it so she's throwing it back on you. Smart woman."

"Thanks. I haven't much time, my hikers are appearing. So what's available?"

"It should be on a weekend, Friday or Saturday evening to draw the most crowd. Tell me when you're free and we'll go from there."

"Shee-e-e," Ramon drew out his hiss through his teeth. Obviously looking at his blotter, he said, "The only weekend I have free between now and November is the weekend after Labor Day and that's just the Friday."

"It looks like that's the date, then. You call her or me?" Roger asked. "Since your hikers are coming, I'll be glad to."

A tiny green jealousy varmint raised its head and waved a tiny flag in front of the handsome young man. "I will!" Ramon swallowed then grumbled fiercely. "Wouldn't want the next most handsome bachelor to crowd me out." Ramon had to grin at his own version of a joke, but of course, Roger didn't see it.

"The *next*...we aren't conceited or anything, are we?"

"Absolutely not! Gotta go!" Ramon could hear chuckling as he replaced the receiver and made a face at it.

He hadn't even removed his hand from the receiver when the door opened and the man said, "Hello, my good man!"

Ramon nodded, as he picked up the receiver again and said, "I'll be with you folks in a minute. Gotta make this call first."

He finished dialing and the voice he heard in his dreams and wanted to hear every day for the rest of his life said a cheery, "Hello!"

"Hi, Sandy talked with Roger and he said it'd have to be the Friday evening after Labor Day. Does that work for you?"

"It does if you're there!"

"That's my only Friday night free all month," he grumbled.

"Great! I'll be ready. How long a concert?"

They hadn't talked about that. He'd never thought. "How about the same as that other concert you gave? Would that work?"

"Sure! I'll have an extra or two just in case, though."

"Super! My office is filling up, I gotta run."

"Have a great one!" Sandy exclaimed. "Oh, if it rains, try dodging between the drops!" She chuckled, as she put down her receiver.

"Mmm, sure," he muttered.

Ramon also put down the receiver and looked up at the dozen people crowded around his desk. "Hi, folks, are you all ready?"

The leader shrugged. "As ready as we can be. Some of us have never been hiking before, so they're a bit apprehensive as well as excited."

Ramon looked around at the group, made up mostly of late teens and smiled. "We'll try to make it a good event for you so you'll feel comfortable by the time we get back. Everyone has a place to sleep inside, away from mosquitoes and has some kind of rain gear? You know we do get showers and rain storms this time of year."

"Yes, we counted tents and we've got enough for everyone to sleep under cover. We really need those?"

"Yes! This time of year the mosquitoes are in full parade form waiting for some sleeping soul to pounce on."

"Great!" one woman grumbled. "I've been mosquito bate all my life."

Another man chuckled and pointed to the young woman who had commented. "That's why we brought Charlotte along with us. Her dad said he always took her fishing, even though she never caught any fish. He's told me she was their best mosquito bate in three counties." He shrugged, "I didn't know and she wanted to come..."

The young, pretty girl swatted the man and said, "Why you! I'll get you for that! Mosquito bate, I'm sure. My dad never said that!"

The man grinned. "Sure he did! Said it right to me."

Ramon nodded at the easy banter and said, "Okay, let's load up and get out of here. It's about that time and we need to get on the move if we want to get anywhere today."

Ramon's pack and tent were beside the door. Everyone trouped out and the door closed. His notepad was in front of him and he looked at the blank page. "Sandy," he wrote, "Have a good week, I'll be back about supper time on Thursday." He almost added, 'Love,' but then wrote, 'Ramon,' instead. What was his problem? He didn't love her! He barely knew her, she was his receptionist; you didn't mix employer/employee relations with pleasure! Right? Right!

He threw down the pen and bolted from behind the desk. Before he could think of anything else to say to her, he grabbed up his backpack, slid his arms through the straps and opened the door. He pushed the lock on the knob and let the door close behind him. He was out of there and wouldn't think of his receptionist while he was on the trail. Piece of cake! *Yeah, right!* that little voice muttered from his shoulder. There had to be lint on his shoulder, he brushed it off.

That evening, when they set up camp, the leader said, "Men, we'll set up the tents while the ladies get the meal. That way, we won't have to eat in the dark."

A teenaged girl sighed, "Division of labor... again."

Ramon set about his favorite job of building the bonfire, and soon the ladies had their meal sizzling over it. The aromas were enticing, especially to Ramon. That's when he remembered he hadn't eaten lunch. When everyone had a plate full and was sitting around the circle, Charlotte said, "Pastor, are you gonna say grace?"

He was the last to sit down and said, "Yes, I'd planned to. Let's bow our heads. Father in heaven, do bless this food to our bodies. Give us a wonderful time on this hike and give us safety. Bless our leader as he directs our way. In Your Son's name, amen."

Again, Ramon thought. The man had prayed for him, even though he didn't do God, never had and never would. He looked at all the people in the group. They raised their heads and dug into their food. They looked normal and they'd acted normal the whole afternoon. The only thing he realized that was different was that he hadn't heard any cussing or bad language since they'd started and one guy had fallen down and skinned up his hand. He hadn't said a word, only wiped off the dirt on his jeans. Just like someone else he knew would do. *You weren't going to think about her, remember?* Ramon scowled and took a big mouthful of stew.

"So who's doing devotions this evening?" the pastor asked.

Now that made Ramon nervous. Devotions? Did he have to sit there and listen to this preacher spout off about God or something? He stuffed another large mouthful into his mouth, not wanting to say anything if someone asked his opinion. He looked from one of the young people to another, then back to the slightly older man, whom the girl had called pastor. He looked around for the closest tree maybe he could take a walk without looking too conspicuous.

One of the guys said, "Since it's Sunday, why don't you do it, Pastor?"

Would they do this all week? Ramon wondered silently. The pastor nodded. "Okay, I will tonight, but you folks be prepared, I'll call on somebody for tomorrow. I'll tell you either when I get finished tonight or first thing in the morning so you'll have all day to think about it."

By the time they'd finished eating, the color was gone from the sky. It was dark, the moon hadn't come up, but there were a million stars. For this meal they'd used disposable plates, cups and silverware and from their places, they tossed them all on the fire. Ramon wasn't too happy about it, but he didn't correct them, they didn't want to lug a bag of trash for five days.

When they were sitting around the fire that was blazing nicely, Ramon forgot he planned to go for a walk and stayed with the group. The pastor pulled out his small Bible and a personal flashlight and said, as he opened the Bible, "I don't know about you folks, but I've been in awe of these hills and the majesty we see at each turn we've made. It brings a Psalm to mind and I think I'll read it to you. It's Psalm 8:

'O LORD, our Lord, how majestic is your name in all the earth!
You have set your glory above the heavens.
From the lips of children and infants you have ordained praise because of your enemies, to silence the foe and the avenger.
When I consider your heavens, the work of your fingers, the moon and the stars which you have set in place, what is man that you are mindful of him, the son of man that you care for him?
You made him a little lower than the heavenly beings and crowned him with glory and honor.
You made him ruler over the works of your hands, you put everything under his feet: all flocks and herds, and the beasts of the field, the birds of the air and the fish of the sea, all that swim the paths of the sea.
O LORD, our Lord, how majestic is your name in all the earth!'

"We have an awesome God, don't we?"

For the first time in his life that he could remember, Ramon looked up at the heavens and saw them in a new perspective. His eyes found some movement in the heavens, a shooting star started at one side of the vast heavens and streaked across to the other. He was awestruck by the beauty of it, of the other stars that provided the background for that one point of light as it moved. This God that he'd been ignoring and pushing out of his life all his life had made all those millions of stars? Each one of them had a place because He'd ordained it? He'd made man? Given him power over all other creatures? This was powerful stuff, it was mind boggling!

He didn't hear too much else that the pastor said, because another thought flew into his mind. Sandy was never far from his thoughts, even though he'd vowed she would not be and a question settled into his mind. If this God was so powerful that he could make all the stars, Man and give him power over every creature on earth, why had He left Sandy without the use of her legs? So the nurse dropped her, if this God was so powerful, why couldn't He have fixed that? He shrugged, no harm in asking this man who was supposed to know the answers about God.

He raised his hand and motioned to the man. Nodding, the pastor asked, "Yes, Ramon, did you want to add something?"

Shaking his head, he said, "I've never been one to believe in these things, but I have a question." The man nodded, but didn't say anything, so Ramon asked, "My receptionist believes in your God, but she has never walked. She is paralyzed from her waist down. If this God you read about is so awesome and powerful, why didn't He fix her when this happened?"

"I can't answer your question completely, Ramon, but God is awesome and powerful, He can do things that we humans can't do. He made our bodies to do awesome things and in many cases they do fix themselves, but some of the parts that He made, He made in such a way that if they are broken or removed or severed, they will not heal or grow back. Yes, He could have performed a miracle, but with her, He chose not to.

"Let me make something clear here. We humans have only one purpose to be here on this earth. We are here to bring glory to God.

When this accident happened to your receptionist, God saw that He would get more glory from her handicap than if she had the use of all her extremities. I know that sounds harsh and unforgiving, but God's ways are far above ours and He sees from the beginning of our lives to the end, in a flash, it is all known to Him."

Ramon dropped his head. He didn't understand why the beautiful, vivacious and happy young woman whom he had come to care so much for should be stuck in a wheelchair all her life just because God didn't think it was necessary to make her well. After all, it was when she was a newborn wouldn't it have been easier to fix it then than if it had happened when she was older?

Ramon had set up his tent after he'd built the fire for the ladies, but tonight he lingered around the fire long after the others found their tents. There hadn't been many mosquitoes buzzing while they sat around the fire, it hadn't rained in a few days. There weren't even many moths flitting around the fire. It was an exceptionally peaceful night.

When everyone was in a tent and finally settled down, Ramon went to his tent and pulled out his sleeping bag. He didn't think he'd be sleeping right away and he wanted to look at the stars while he thought. They were so awesome tonight. Finally, the moon came up and shed some cold light on the quiet scene around him.

There were no clouds, only the millions of stars and the crescent moon that at first was a bright orange on the horizon, but then became silver as it worked its way higher into the black velvet sky. It was awesome whoever had written those words was probably looking at a sky like this. He put his hands under his head, enjoying the silence. He felt himself getting sleepy, so he got up from his sleeping bag and dragged it into his tent, then crawled into his bag and closed his eyes. If the problem hadn't been solved in twenty-five years, he wasn't likely to solve it tonight.

Sandy hung up from talking to Ramon about the concert. She wondered why she'd consented she'd hated that time in Philly and been really nervous. Most of those people she'd known. There were only a few people in Vansville that she knew, and this church wasn't her home church. She'd never met the pastor, didn't know what he looked like. All she knew about him was his first name was Roger and he sometimes hiked with Ramon. Not much to go on, really. She wondered why, if Isabel was right, why such a man became a minister. If he didn't have any more to talk about than something like a Reader's Digest article, what was the point?

She guessed it didn't matter she had a concert to prepare for, an hour and a half concert to be exact! She went to the piano and began going through her repertoire. She'd love to play the pieces she loved and could play from memory, but that would be no challenge. Hadn't she always made a point to expand her horizons every chance she could? She set several of her favorites aside with a sigh and picked up one of her books, glad that Ed had sent them along then looked through her sheet music. One piece she'd always considered a challenge, but had never tackled it stood out of the pack. She opened the sheet music to the first page. She must go through this one hand at a time. There were a lot of intricate places that would need special work if she planned to play it perfectly. At a concert anything but perfection was not an option. Chopin was not one you ran over roughshod, either. The masters wrote their music to be played a certain way and anyone who did so must follow directions.

When suppertime came, she was tired, but it was a good tired, she'd completed the entire piece, hands separately. Another day she'd tackle putting the hands together, then when she had that under her belt, she'd start her metronome and bring it gradually up to speed. This would be her major work for the concert, she'd fill in the rest of the time with things she knew and loved.

Later, as she lay in bed, she wondered how many children would come. If she had her way, most of her students would be children. She smiled, one day soon, she'd find her book that had Mozart's piece that people knew as 'Twinkle, Twinkle Little Star' and brush up on that. Every child knew:

'Twinkle, twinkle little star, how I wonder what you are.
Up above the world so high, like a diamond in the sky.
Twinkle, twinkle little star, how I wonder what you are.'

Sandy looked out her window. After she turned out the light, she always looked out the window close by. Tonight there were millions of stars. She knew the moon was up, but she couldn't see it from her bed. Ramon was out there somewhere. Was he in his tent, in his sleeping bag? Had he looked up at the stars? Did he realize or even think about the fact that God had made every one? even had a name for it?

She closed her eyes and opened her heart in prayer. "God, my Father, You know Ramon's heart. You know he wasn't raised in a Christian home as I was. He seems completely opposed to everything I say that even mentions You. He told me this was a church group he was leading this week. May something that is said touch his heart, open it, I pray to You. Let him realize his need for You and Your gift to make him a new person through the shed blood of Your Son. I pray in His name, Amen."

Sandy rarely listened to the radio and never the TV. She had too many interests in other things to be bothered to turn on the tube. However, when she woke up on Wednesday morning, the clouds hung low and heavy over Vansville. Tuesday had been a beautiful day, the temperature had been about right for the end of August, but there had been a breeze that seemed to come from those hills that Ramon loved so much. However, Wednesday was totally opposite. There was no sun the clouds were so thick at dawn that no colors had appeared. Overnight the breeze had stiffened to a downright cold wind and Sandy was glad for the well insulated cabin, as she looked out the window. The trees were whipping around. This wouldn't be a nice day at all to be on the trail, whether they were coming back or not.

As Sandy left for Ramon's office, Isabel was puttering in her flower bed at her front step. "Hi, Isabel!" Sandy called, as she turned the key to open the big door. "It's not a nice day, is it?"

"No, Missy, it's not nice at all. The first hurricane of the season is blowing up along the coast from Florida. We're supposed to get rain starting this afternoon and by tonight it'll be really upon us. Back inland like this, we don't get the terrible winds, but we do get lots of rain. Sometimes it even floods between here and Blairsville, but not near what they get on the coast."

Scowling, Sandy asked, "What happens to Ramon and his group? They're not scheduled to get back until tomorrow evening."

Isabel shrugged. "He'll probably try to find them a place that's protected. There are lots of groves that they can camp overnight in. They'll have to get wet while they hike. That's one of the hazards of hiking around here."

"I guess, but rain can make a day so dismal."

"Do you have to go to his place today?"

"Yes, I'm there from nine to twelve."

"I'm afraid you'll get wet if you stay that long."

Sandy shrugged. "I've been wet before. I haven't melted yet, so I doubt I will this time, either. See you, Isabel."

"Yes, Missy. Take care."

She waved and wheeled herself onto the lift. "I'll do my best."

Ramon crawled from his tent Wednesday morning to a leaden sky. He'd heard on Sunday that a tropical storm was in the Atlantic, close to Puerto Rico. Perhaps it had become a hurricane that was now coming up the coast. It was a bit early for a hurricane, but there was always an exception. Weather conditions were right. He shrugged, he knew where they'd need to camp tonight, but they'd still be in rain all day tomorrow if that was the case. Camping in the rain was not his favorite thing to do, but it couldn't be helped sometimes. He always told the person who contacted him to make sure the hikers had raingear.

He rattled the leader's tent support and called, "Hey, folks, we need to get on the trail. I think we're in for some dismal weather that'll give us rain before we're back to your vehicles."

There were a lot of groans and then tents started moving as their occupants began getting ready for the day. Ramon had to hand it to these guys, they hadn't complained about anything and they didn't this morning, either. As the day went on, the wind picked up and by evening, in the grove, they could hear it whistling in the tops of the trees.

He looked at the regular cooks as he led them into the trees and asked, "Do you ladies have a cold menu for this evening? I think we'd better do without a fire tonight. Not only are we in the trees, but the wind is pretty strong and could whip a fire out of our control pretty fast."

"Yes, we'll figure something out, Ramon."

That evening, there was no bonfire, but they did have devotions, just as they'd had each night. It was the pastor's turn and as before, Ramon had nothing else to do, so he sat with the group to hear what the man had to say. Again this evening, he pulled out his little Bible and his flashlight. "Folks, I want to read my favorite Psalm to you tonight. I may not do much else, but these verses have a powerful message all by themselves. Listen to Psalm 139."

"'O LORD, you have searched me and you know me.
You know when I sit and when I rise; you perceive my thoughts from afar.
You discern my going out and my lying down;
you are familiar with all my ways.
Before a word is on my tongue you know it completely, O LORD.
You hem me in - behind and before; you have laid your hand upon me.
Such knowledge is too wonderful for me, too lofty for me to attain.
Where can I go from your Spirit?
Where can I flee from your presence?
If I go up to the heavens, you are there; if I make my bed in the
depths, you are there.
If I rise on the wings of the dawn, if I settle on the far side of the sea,
even there your hand will guide me, your right hand will hold me fast.
If I say, "Surely the darkness will hide me and the light become night
around me," even the darkness will not be dark to you; the night will
shine like the day, for darkness is as light to you.
For you created my inmost being; you knit me together in my
mother's womb.
I praise you because I am fearfully and wonderfully made; your works
are wonderful, I know that full well.
My frame was not hidden from you when I was made in the secret place.
When I was woven together in the depths of the earth, your eyes saw
my unformed body.
All the days ordained for me were written in your book before
one of them came to be.
How precious to me are your thoughts, O God! How vast
is the sum of them!

Were I to count them, they would outnumber the grains of sand.
When I awake, I am still with you.
If only you would slay the wicked, O God!
Away from me, you bloodthirsty men!
They speak of you with evil intent; your adversaries misuse your name.
Do I not hate those who hate you, O Lord, and abhor those who rise
up against you?
I have nothing but hatred for them; I count them my enemies.
Search me, O God, and know my heart; test me and know
my anxious thoughts.
See if there is any offensive way in me, and lead me
in the way everlasting.'"
Psalm 139

The leader didn't say anything else, but one of the young men voiced Ramon's thoughts exactly when he murmured, "Awesome!"

After several others made some comments and the leader closed their session with prayer, Ramon said, "I hate to come down to something so practical, but we must be on the move early in the morning. I'm sure it'll be raining soon and perhaps it'll rain all day tomorrow. If it does, the trails will be muddy and in some places very slippery. That'll slow us down a lot, so if we want to get back before dark tomorrow, we'll have to move as fast as we can. However, it's also imperative that we move as carefully as we can, too, because mud can do terrible things to progress. It knows no friends and we must be constantly aware. Sleep well!"

Ramon was the last to climb in his tent. He made it a habit to do that to be sure everyone was accounted for. These teens seemed responsible, but they had paid him good money and he'd make sure he fulfilled his part. He had barely zipped down the tent flaps when the first drop fell on his tent. He wondered if the others had made sure they and their belongings were away from the sides of their tents to keep them from letting water in. He shrugged and closed his eyes. He couldn't be mother to all of his hikers they had to take some responsibility for themselves.

During the night he woke up to the rain pounding down on his tent. He wasn't wet and he knew they were high enough that there was no chance of flooding, but he wondered about the trails they still must travel. The last trail they must take to reach his parking lot crossed a stream and it was known to flood occasionally. It hadn't rained in a few days, but this was really coming down, would it be enough to flood the stream? It was dark, very dark under the trees. He pressed the button on his watch and it showed him that the time was four o'clock. He hoped he'd wake at first light, they'd need to be on the trail as early as possible, rain or not.

He turned over, but the last verse the pastor read came to him. 'Search me, O God, and know my heart; test me and know my anxious thoughts. See if there is any offensive way in me, and lead me in the way everlasting.' Psalm 139: 23,24. Could God do that? Could He know his heart, his thoughts? Could he see things in him that were offensive? He shivered, but not because he was cold. These were heavy thoughts, ones that he'd never thought before. His mother surely hadn't fostered any thoughts about God. He'd always thought that God was some far off thing, that is, if there was such a thing at all. According to what the pastor read from his Bible both times, God wasn't far off He was close enough and interested enough to know his every thought. If that was true, it was a scary thought!

Ramon drifted off to sleep again and in a little over an hour he woke up. A hint of light turned the green of his tent from forest green to grass green. He heard the rain, it hadn't stopped, in fact, it was coming down hard and the wind was still whipping the trees over them. He slithered from his sleeping bag and rolled it up, then stuffed it into its waterproof bag. Quickly he pulled his rain slicker over his head, then left the tent, found a tree to relieve himself and rattled the leader's tent.

"Rise and shine, folks! It's morning and we need to be on the way soon."

"I hear you, Ramon," A sleepy voice said.

He went back to his tent, took it down quickly and shook off the water, then quickly folded it and put it in its travel bag. He'd lay it out in the laundry when he got home. Everyone hurried with their morning routines, ate the granola bars the ladies came up with and were set to leave before seven. Some rain drops made it through the trees, but when they left the grove, they were pelted with water.

"How far is it back to your place?" the pastor asked.

"We'll be lucky to get there by supper time. I've never worn a pedometer, so I can't say for sure, but probably five miles, but with the rain and muddy trails it'll seem like more."

"Great," Charlotte muttered. "I could go for a nice, warm, **dry** gym right now, I wouldn't mind even if I had to exercise."

When Sandy woke up she looked out her window and saw the rain coming in rivers down her window. The trees beyond were swaying majestically, then she shivered. She had a rain slicker, but if she covered herself with it, it left her chair vulnerable and the battery didn't work well when it got wet. If she put the slicker over her head and let much of it go over the back of the chair to cover the battery, her legs and feet got wet. Perhaps she could take a garbage bag and cover her lap and as far as it would go down her legs. It hardly mattered she'd be wet to some degree when she reached the office.

She had a feeling she needed to be there and maybe needed to stay later than noon. She shrugged she'd do what she had to do. She drank a cup of coffee for breakfast, knowing she needed to be as warm as possible to ward off the chill of being wet. Ramon had cocoa and if she felt the need, she could fix herself a cup of hot chocolate at his place. When she went out on her porch it didn't feel like August at all. The wind was whipping around and the cold rain made it feel like the end of October or even November. She shivered and hurried to the van. Of course, the controls wouldn't be hurried they opened at the appointed speed. In Ramon's parking lot it was the reverse and Sandy was soaked as she wheeled herself to the office door. She went inside and quickly shed her rain slicker and the big garbage bag, draping them over a chair.

Ramon and his group started out, going as quickly as they could for the conditions. Later on, he noticed that everyone was concentrating on putting one foot ahead of the other and keeping up with his pace. He was going as fast as he dared. There was a hill made up of shale that they must cross, it would be the most treacherous part of their hike unless the stream was over its banks. Before lunch they reached the hill of shale that they must descend. There was no going around it.

Ramon stopped the group and when everyone was gathered, he said, "We've come to the worst part of the trail. In good weather it's hard to cross, but with the rain and wet hiking boots we must be even more careful."

He looked around for the pastor and said, "Would you please go down first, then wait at the bottom. Be as careful as you can and take as much time as you need. I'll watch for you and then send each one as I think they should go."

The older man looked ahead and saw the shale, but he asked Ramon, "Would it be all right if I prayed before we tackle this?"

"Of course, it's fine."

Everyone took hands and included Ramon in their circle. He felt a little strange, he'd never prayed in his life, but he closed his eyes along with everyone else. The pastor said, "Father, we place ourselves in Your hands. Ramon says this is the most dangerous part of our hike and I know he's right. Father, we don't expect the rain to stop, but do protect us and keep us in the palm of Your hand. Thank You, Amen."

The pastor started out and inched his way down the shifting, slippery slope. Ramon watched him, keeping the others away from the shale on the grass on top. When the pastor was part way down, Ramon said to the oldest teen, "You go now and when you get to where he is now, you stop. I'll position you men along the trail so you can help those who come after you. I'll bring up the rear."

The young man set out and before he reached his station, the pastor reached the bottom. Ramon sent two more men to positions along the trail and finally started sending the women. The fourth woman didn't have hiking boots. Ramon had been concerned about her all along, since all she had were tennis shoes. She'd done fine until the rain. He sent her with a buddy, he didn't want to take any chances with her. He held the last two women back until the two were nearly to the pastor, but when he turned his back, he heard a scream. He whirled around and one of the women was crumpled on the shale. Even from where he stood on top, he could see that her leg was in an unnatural position. She would have to be transported out. How would he manage that? None of these people had ever been on this trail before. He was so intent on assessing the situation he forgot about the cold rain using his hair as a runway to his neck.

One of the women still beside him said, "Ramon, do you have a cell phone?"

He made a face and said, "No, I don't. Before I head out again I will have one!" he vowed. "She will need transporting, someone will have to hike out and call."

The woman worked her backpack from her back, then found a side pocket and pulled out a cell phone. "If we can get reception, we can call from here."

Ramon breathed a sigh and said, "From up here we should be able to connect with the towers or satellite from Blairsville."

"Who can you call? Is there a 911 available?"

"No, I'll have to call Sandy she should still be at my office."

"Great! God is good!" she exclaimed.

Is He? The woman broke her leg! Ramon mused.

At ten till twelve the phone rang. Sandy answered, "DeLord's Hiking and Camp....."

Ramon's voice broke in; he had only one thought, so he said, "Sandy! I'm so glad you're there! I'm using a hiker's cell phone. We've had an injury and we need an airlift. Call the Blairsville Hospital and ask for Fisher. He's with MEDIVAC. I'll give you this cell phone number so you can pass it on. They'll have to call me so I can give them the location."

Sandy took down the directions and the number and said, "It's not you, is it, Ramon?"

"No, it's one of the girls and she's hurt quite badly. The pastor's staying with her and I'm bringing the rest out. We should be there about five o'clock if nothing else happens. This trail is awful! Thanks, Sandy, glad you're there!"

They disconnected and Sandy followed Ramon's instructions to the letter. As soon as she hung up from talking to Dr. Fisher, she began to pray. She never thought to leave the office, she even forgot to fix any lunch for herself, even though there was food in Ramon's refrigerator she could have eaten. At four o'clock, she finally looked at the clock on the desk and remembered that Ramon had said he'd be back around five. She didn't know where any more phones were, so she took the portable one from Ramon's desk and went down the hall to the kitchen. She looked through his cupboards and in his refrigerator and decided she would make him supper. He needed a hot meal after being out in this all day. Soon there was a wonderful aroma going throughout the whole house, as the contents of the pans simmered on the stove.

When he hung up from talking to Sandy, he said to the two women, "Start down, I'll need to stay here until they call from MEDIVAC. Tell the men to follow you and then tell the pastor he'll need to stay with our injured lady until they come."

Only moments later the phone in his hand rang, quickly, he said, "Ramon DeLord."

"Ramon, it's Len with MEDIVAC. You need transport?"

He swallowed a sigh that wanted to escape and said, "Yes, I'm glad it's you, Len. We're doing this shale mountain and I've got an obvious fracture of a large leg bone. I know you know where we are. I'm leaving a man with the injured, but since it's raining so hard, I'll lead the rest of the group out."

"I'll be there as soon as I can. Take extra care. I don't know for sure, but I'll bet anything that stream ahead of you's climbing its banks."

Ramon nodded and said on a sigh, "I've been thinking that, too. I think you're right. We'll be careful, Len and thanks."

"No problem."

Ramon closed the phone and looked down the side of the mountain. The two women had passed the first man who followed them closely. Ramon started down, but moved cautiously, he didn't want to loosen any of the shale with his hiking boots and send it down onto those in front of him. He could hear the injured woman moaning from the place where she'd fallen.

The pastor had helped the woman's partner down and she joined the others at the bottom, but then he'd climbed back up the short ways and helped the injured woman remove her backpack, then helped her cover her head with her rain slicker. He stayed with her, shielding her as best he could with his body. Finally, the two women reached the bottom and along with them the men who had held their positions. Ramon was the only one left on the shale.

When he reached the injured woman and the pastor, he said, "Thank goodness Charlotte had her cell phone and I was able to call out! The MEDIVAC knows where you are. He's hiked with me before and knows this area quite well. Hopefully, he can land his chopper over there where the group is standing and airlift you both out. He'll have room for your packs, too. I think the best thing is to leave you two here and I'll take the rest of the group on to base. Shall I leave you with the cell phone?"

"If he knows where we are, we should be okay. God forbid, but you may need it again. Take it with you." He turned to the rest of the group and in his pulpit voice, he said, "I'll call Ramon's office from wherever the chopper takes us. Ramon'll get you back safely, I'm sure."

The group hadn't been very vocal all day, it was hard to speak over the rain and wind when they were going single file. Now that they had to leave their leader and a member of their group in the rain by themselves, they were even more subdued.

They fell in line behind Ramon, but hadn't gone far when they all heard the distinctive thumping of helicopter blades. In fact, the bird went over them first before it settled on the wet ground behind them. Ramon sighed, but didn't speak.

The injured woman's partner sighed and said, "Thank goodness! I'm glad they didn't have to wait too long. This rain is so depressing."

Ramon gave the woman's phone back and said, "I'm to lead another group tomorrow, but if they haven't called to cancel, I'll call them. Even if it stops raining before you leave, it'll be too wet to go on these trails for several days. At any rate, now that I know one'll work out in these mountains, by tomorrow night I'll have an activated cell phone that I'll carry every time. Thanks for having yours and letting me use it."

The woman nodded and slipped the phone in a pocket. "We've found they pay for themselves, especially with kids. We've had two cars leave their drivers stranded and they've had to call us. At first you think it's a terrible expense, but soon you realize it isn't. I'm sure glad I had it and that it worked out here on the trail."

"I definitely agree!"

Sandy was in Ramon's kitchen fixing supper when the phone rang. Her heart jumped into her throat, as she pulled it from beside her and answered. She didn't know the voice and she was momentarily disappointed. The voice said, "Hello, Ma'am, this is Pastor Eldon, has Ramon reached the office yet?"

"No, sir, I haven't heard from him since he called about sending a MEDIVAC to pick up someone who was injured. Is everything all right?"

"We've arrived at the Dalton Hospital. The pilot was kind enough to bring us all the way here, since this is our home town. Tell my people when they arrive that we're both okay and that they should pack up their things in the cars and drive home. We both have family who have already come. Marjorie's leg has been set, but they're keeping her overnight for observation."

"I'll be sure to tell everyone that you called and give them the message."

TEN

"Sandy, is it?" the pastor continued, "Tell Ramon thanks for the great time we've had. I think we'll want to go again next year, but I'll have to call later about that."

"Thanks, Rev. Eldon, I'll be sure he knows. I'm sorry there was a mishap, but at least it was on the last day on the way back."

"Yes, that's true and it wouldn't have happened if it hadn't been raining, I'm sure. Thanks again for everything."

"You're welcome."

Sandy sighed with relief, but no one was back. The pot of chili was simmering when she heard noise in the office. She wheeled herself down the hall, but had never seen so many bedraggled people before. However, she only had eyes for Ramon. He was as wet as the rest, but she hardly noticed, she couldn't believe how glad she was to see them all, but especially him. Ramon was at his desk when Sandy came through the doorway from the rest of the house.

He looked up and momentarily, he was speechless, just looking at her. He swallowed and asked, "Has anyone called?"

"Yes, only moments ago the pastor called to say they'd been evacuated to Dalton. He said to load up and go on home, there's no need to worry about them, they're in good hands. The lady is staying in the hospital over night."

A young man a little older than Ramon said, "I guess we're out of here! Thanks, Ramon, thanks for a great time and thanks for keeping your head in this."

Ramon held out his hand and the two men shook. "Rob, I'm sorry it happened, but I'm glad I have the kind of backup I do. You all drive safely, it's a ways to Dalton. You've had quite a day and the rain doesn't look like it's about to let up any time soon."

"It's not," Sandy said. "We're getting the full brunt of the first hurricane of the season. It's supposed to rain and be strong winds for three days."

"Oh, great!" Ramon and two others grumbled.

While everyone was shaking hands with Ramon and heading out the door, the phone rang. Sandy answered again and the voice said, "I need to speak to Ramon DeLord, please."

"I'm sorry, he's busy right now, could I answer your questions or would you prefer I take a message to have him call you?"

"You'll see him before tomorrow?"

"Yes, sir, probably before half an hour is up."

"Tell him Lewis Marchant called. I'm the leader for tomorrow's three day hike. I think the hurricane's done us a number and we'd better take our lumps and stay home."

Sandy laughed. "I'm with you on that! Stay home and dry."

She hung up as Ramon walked back in the office, as car doors slammed and shook his head. "It's a rainy night in Georgia."

Giving him her perpetual smile, she said, "Yes, and you're soaked. There's probably not a dry inch on you! Get dried off I've got a pot full of chili simmering on the stove waiting for you to come eat it."

"You don't know how good that sounds, Sandy!"

"I thought it might."

Tomorrow started Labor Day weekend. Ramon had been looking forward to this hike most of the summer, because these were friends and acquaintances that he'd hiked with before and who had graduated from the normal trails to the more rugged, less traveled trails that he loved but didn't get to go on very often. However, now that it was here, he wasn't. Sandy had entered his life and no matter how much he told himself she was his employee, his heart didn't believe a word of it. His brain had finally believed what his ears heard her say several times that she didn't plan to leave Vansville when his job for her was finished. He guessed he'd hoped all along that she wouldn't, but he didn't understand why she was staying around.

Sandy left at noon, as she normally did, but Duncan Roads was scheduled to come by about three this afternoon. Ramon had lots of things to go over with him he hoped he could spend more time on the trails with him before the end of October so he could become familiar with the area before their season started again in the spring.

The light blue van had left the parking lot, so Ramon tore his eyes away from the last spot where he'd seen it. He stood up and stretched, then went to his kitchen and fixed some sandwiches for lunch. He brought them and a huge glass of iced tea back to his office. He needed to get his thoughts and supplies together before Duncan arrived. Usually, the groups who came were friends and he expected them to supply their own food, plus enough for him. These people were all friends of his, but weren't coming as a group together, so he had planned to supply the food. It had been a big undertaking. All the food, regular food and dried packages, were piled in one chair in the office.

Ramon was tall, six foot two inches with light olive skin that reflected his Latin heritage. His eyes and hair were dark brown and his hair was a little long, but he liked it that way, besides, he was his own person. He did shave at least he did when he was home. On the trail it grew, he didn't take a razor. Because of his hiking, he was very much in shape and even in the winter when he wasn't hiking, he walked around town a lot. He liked to be outside and to walk. Vansville was just the right size to take in in an hour's walk.

However, the man who stepped from the SUV at three o'clock was quite different. Perhaps the only things about him that were similar to Ramon was that he was tall and well built. Duncan was fair skinned, but had a deep tan, his hair was blond and hung down his back in a ponytail and when he entered Ramon's office, he saw that Duncan had a blond beard brushing his chest and his eyes were a startling blue. The man was dressed already as if he was planning to leave for a hike momentarily in hiking boots, jeans and a plaid, button down shirt, all that was missing was the backpack. Ramon was sure it was already packed and in the back of his SUV.

He pushed the door open and entered the office with his hand out. A smile split the hair on his face and his eyes sparkled. He strode across the space and in a rich baritone, he said, "Afternoon! I'm Duncan Roads; I presume you're Ramon DeLord? I sure am happy to meet you!" his voice boomed around the room.

Matching his smile, Ramon held out his hand and grasped Duncan's in a firm shake. "Yes, I am. I'm pleased to meet you, Duncan."

The man looked around the office, Ramon wasn't sure what he was looking for, but he made a thorough inspection, noticing Ramon's photos and Sandy's painting, before he said, "Didn't I speak with a lady named Sandy when I called? Doesn't she work here any longer?"

"Yes," Ramon tried to keep his voice neutral, even though he could feel a green monster sitting on his shoulder. "Sandy still works here, but she's only here in the morning. She takes care of everything that's needed in three hours." *Thank goodness!*

Duncan nodded, but asked, "Perhaps she'll be here in the morning? I want to thank her for passing on my message."

Ramon shook his head. "No, she's only here five days a week and I gave her Monday off, since it's the holiday." Wanting to change the subject, Ramon asked, "Do you have hiking and camping equipment?"

Duncan thumbed his fist over his shoulder, and said, "Sure! I've hiked and camped for many years. I even have my laptop in my car and I've scoped out these hills and mountains on the web, so I'm a bit familiar with the area. Of course, there's nothing like tramping the real thing, so I'm anxious to be on the trails tomorrow. You said this was a scheduled hike, how many will go with us?"

"Actually, there will be six of us altogether and we'll leave at eight o'clock. Where will you stay for the night?"

"Since you said there are no motels here in Vansville, I took a room in Blairsville. I'll need to eat before I arrive, is that right?"

"Yes, that's why I make eight o'clock the time we leave from base so people will have eaten breakfast before they come. Since you'll be going along as a new guide, would you like to come for breakfast so we can look at the map together first? Are you a coffee drinker? You look like the type who could put food away well."

"Sure, that'll be great! I'll bring my laptop in and program it in."

Ramon felt at a disadvantage, since he'd never used a computer for his hikes, or even thought about doing so. Curious, he asked, "Do you carry your laptop on a trail?"

Duncan shrugged. "There's a slot for one on my backpack, but often I print out a copy to take, it's not as heavy, but the laptop shows things in 3D, so it's easier to know the rough spots."

"I see that might be something you can help me with. Will you be staying in the area during the off season?"

The blond giant grinned. "I don't really have a place I call 'home,' I can stay in the area or go somewhere else. What did you have in mind?"

Ramon nodded at his office in general and said, "As you can see, I have no computer, Sandy takes the calls and records them on my calendar here and in my appointment book. I've thought about getting a computer, but it's never happened. Perhaps if you stayed in the area over the winter, we could set up something like that and maybe expand some, each of us taking a trip occasionally. Sandy says she's staying in the area permanently, so I could probably persuade her to help us out some." *Now why did I say that? Don't I want to keep her for myself?*

"Sure! You said there are no motels in town, are there places to be rented?"

Without any hesitation, he said, "There's a row of cabins on the far edge of town that the lady rents by the month, but that can be rented indefinitely if someone wants to. That's my only suggestion." What was he doing? *Clunk me over the head with a bat!* If he wasn't careful, he'd be throwing Duncan at Sandy! He wasn't a *real* dunce, was he?

Duncan shrugged. "I'm good with that."

While Ramon and Duncan discussed the hike for the next day, the phone rang. Ramon didn't answer his phone any more when he had someone there, so he let it ring and the machine picked up. On the other end came a familiar voice, "Ramon, I had planned to bring four of my paintings with me this morning for you to hang...."

Ramon picked up the receiver and said, "Hi, Sandy! Did you want to bring them over this afternoon? I can hang them now and my hikers tomorrow can see them."

"Would you, Ramon? That is what I wanted, can I come now?"

"Sure, any time this afternoon." At that moment he looked up and saw the interested Duncan watching him and wanted to take back those words he'd said to Sandy, but of course, he held no cords to Sandy, she was still a free woman, so he said, "So when will you be over?"

"It'll take me a few minutes to gather them up, but how about fifteen minutes; will that be okay with you?"

"It'll be fine." He'd introduce his two employees and if there was any attraction between the two of them, then that would let him off the hook, right? *Are you ever thick-headed!* That little voice from his shoulder exclaimed.

"Is that the Sandy who works here?" Duncan asked.

"Yes, she's also an artist. When we first met she painted that picture. I bought it from her and hung it in here." He pointed to the painting that hung prominently on the wall. "Then I told her if she had more I'd let her use this room as a gallery if she liked. She's bringing four over." Looking at his photos he said, "I'll need to decide which of my photos to take down."

"Good, I'll get to meet her after all."

"Yes, I guess you will," Ramon grumbled.

Even though Ramon tried to talk about hiking in general and the hike they were going on the next day, he knew that both he and Duncan were distracted, knowing who would be here in only a few minutes. Of course, Duncan had no idea that Sandy sat in a wheelchair. Ramon wondered what his first reaction would be. He hoped the man wouldn't treat her as his mom did. He'd probably dismiss him immediately.

Right on time, the blue van turned onto his parking lot and pulled into her regular place. Ramon could see the side where she left the van and he raised his head to watch. Duncan noticed that Ramon had stopped talking, so he turned to see the van stop. He looked back at the map that Ramon had pulled out, but then looked back outside when he didn't hear a car door slam. What he saw was the door sliding open and a lift slowly descend to its horizontal position.

Ramon still watched as the beautiful woman wheeled herself onto the lift, but Duncan gasped and said, "She's handicapped? But she spoke very intelligently to me!"

Ramon glanced back at the man and scowled. "So? Why wouldn't she?"

Duncan waved his hand at the door and said, "But she's handicapped!"

Ramon only had the chance to say, "Yes, her legs don't move, that's all."

Sandy opened the door, as Ramon and Duncan both stood up and wheeled herself inside. She smiled at Ramon, then turned and glanced at Duncan. Instantly, feeling uncomfortable, Sandy said, "Hi, I didn't remember he was coming this afternoon. Here, I'll leave these you hang them wherever you want. I'll...."

"Sandy, meet Duncan Roads. He's going on the hike tomorrow. Duncan, my receptionist, Sandy Bernard."

Duncan nodded, but didn't reach out his hand, instead he swallowed. "Afternoon, pleased to meet you."

Sandy dropped her hand back to her paintings that were on her lap, but with a smile, she said, "Hello, Duncan, I'm pleased to meet you. I hope you and Ramon can come to some agreements, he's been covered up this year and needs some relief." She looked back at Ramon and said, "Will you have room for these? I hate for you to take your wonderful prints down."

Letting out a sigh of frustration, Ramon said, "Sandy, didn't I tell you we'd make a gallery for your paintings?"

She nodded. "Yes, you did, but these prints you have are beautiful."

Ramon came around to behind her chair and said, "Let me see your paintings. I doubt there'll be any contest as to which ones stay or go."

Sandy picked up her first one and put it on the far corner of his desk, then put the second one next, then the third and last of all the fourth. Silently watching as she laid them out, Ramon finally said, "Sandy! These are of that view we saw from that trail! Awesome! Are these from your photos or are they from when you went back?"

Knowing they had a silent audience, she blushed and said, "No, I haven't had time to go back yet, the first two I had finished before I got the pictures back. I made some minor changes after seeing the prints."

Ramon shook his head, still gazing at the beautiful paintings. "There is no contest which ones get hung! Duncan, since you're here, you can help me take these four down and hand me Sandy's paintings to take their places."

Duncan had been busy ever since Sandy entered the room looking first at her, then at her chair, then after she spread out her paintings at them. He swallowed and looked at Ramon as he pulled a straight chair from one side of the room to another corner and said, "Ahh, sure, which one do you want? These are great."

Climbing up on the chair, he took down the first print and said, "That far one, of course, it's the first one of the panorama."

"Sure! I'm with you on that."

Duncan picked up the one that Ramon indicated and held it out with one hand, ready to take the print Ramon handed him. However, Sandy said, "Thanks, so much, Ramon. I'll leave you and Duncan alone and get to my practicing. It's a week from today, you know."

Ramon still stood on the chair when Sandy turned around to go. "Sandy," he said, "don't leave on our account. If I remember right, you don't need much practice to 'play like an angel.'"

She chuckled, sitting in the open doorway. "Come on, Ramon, any musician needs to practice before giving a concert. Don't let anyone fool you." She moved through the doorway and closed the door behind her. Ramon nearly dropped the painting, he hadn't wanted her to leave so soon…. but of course, he did! He had things to do and a new colleague to familiarize with the area. What was he thinking?

As Duncan handed Ramon the second picture, he asked, "She doesn't have to practice her painting, does she? This is first class!"

"No, she'll give a concert next Friday night. I'm surprised she's finished these four paintings so quickly. After I hung that picture of hers, two couples came back and asked her to paint a picture for them. One was a portrait of the couple and the other was from a photo they'd taken on their hike. She had them finished within a week, but now she says she has to practice. I've heard her play I've never heard anything so professional!" Ramon sighed, "She insists I must be the MC for the concert. I hope I don't drop the ball. Give me the great outdoors, I'm not one to stand in front of a crowd!"

"What does she play what instrument? Will she have an accompanist?"

"The piano."

"The... what?"

Ramon climbed down from the chair to move it. As he did, he said, "The piano. She's fantastic! There's none better!"

Duncan shook his head. "No way!"

Ramon nodded and stepped up on the chair again. "Yes. Her landlady says she plays like an angel. I've heard her, she's super!"

"Friday you say? I'll be here!"

As if he'd expected otherwise, Duncan said, "There really isn't anything wrong with her except that her legs don't move! Was she in an accident?"

"She was dropped as a newborn in the hospital nursery," Ramon said, matter-of-factly.

Instantly agitated, Duncan exclaimed, "**What**! Did her parents sue, didn't they try the neurosurgeons? What gives?"

Ramon shrugged. "I don't know, she's never said. That was all she told me and she seemed a bit reluctant to tell me more."

Duncan grumbled something under his breath, but didn't comment out loud.

Ramon stepped from the chair, stood back and said, "There, that's great!"

Sandy truly had forgotten that Duncan was to come this afternoon. She could have kicked herself when she wheeled into the office and saw the man sitting beside Ramon's desk. She hadn't meant to interrupt his meeting with the man she'd only thought to get her pictures up so that his hikers would see them. She knew she wouldn't be in at all this weekend and if they weren't hanging, these hikers wouldn't see them. So far, she hadn't received any calls for piano students. She had sold those paintings to Ramon's hikers, but she knew that shortly she'd need to have some money coming in so she could live through the winter.

She wheeled herself into her cabin and over to the piano. She opened the Chapin piece, then started her metronome and soon let the music she was playing wash over her. She had most of the piece memorized, but it wasn't quite up to speed yet. She had been concentrating on this piece, but she had her program finalized in her mind.

She lifted her hands from the keys for a rest and the phone rang. She sighed, turned off the metronome and wheeled herself to the nearest phone. She needed to get an answering machine, but hadn't had a chance to get back to Blairsville to make the purchase. "Hello?" she said on the third ring.

"Sandy Bernard?"

"Yes, I'm Sandy."

"Sandy, I'm Roger Clemens. I call myself the preacher at the local church. I'm looking at my calendar and realized we have you scheduled for a concert next Friday."

"Yes, Reverend, is that a problem?"

"Please! No reverend for me! I'm Roger to everyone in town. Do you have a list of your pieces you wish to play? Could I get that list and make up a program?"

"Sure! Ramon is the MC, did he tell you that?"

Roger chuckled. "Yes, he told me, quite reluctantly, of course."

"If you'd want to come now I could give you my list. I was practicing, so I'll be here the rest of the afternoon and evening."

"Fine, I'll be right over."

Roger had never seen Sandy, never been around town at the same time. Of course, Ramon had told him a little about her, but he was anxious to meet her face to face. Since there was no parsonage, Roger had built himself a homestead on some property not too far out of town and supplemented his meager income that he received from the church with a small farm. He climbed in his Jeep and left for town and the cabins on the other side of town from the church.

Ramon had told him that Sandy used a wheelchair, but it didn't hit him until he drove onto Isabel's parking lot and saw Sandy's van parked parallel to the drive, that she was in need of a ramp to get into a building. His church had five steps! The back door was no better. Maybe between now and next Friday he'd round up a few men who'd help him build a ramp so she could get from the sidewalk into the church. If she drove a van he assumed she wanted to be as independent as possible. He wondered again how she could play a piano if her legs didn't move, however, there was no denying it she was playing as he walked up.

He walked up her ramp and could hear the most beautiful music coming from the cabin. He didn't go to the door right away, but stood back on the porch for a few minutes. He scowled, if she was in a wheelchair that meant she couldn't walk. Did she somehow have some use of her feet so she could use the sustaining pedal? When she came to a pause, he knocked and she came immediately. She flung open the door and smiled at the young man. His heart turned over at that smile, this was one beautiful woman. No wonder Ramon warned him off!

"Hi, you must be Roger Clemens!"

"Yes, you must be Sandy Bernard," he said, holding out his hand.

She shook his hand, then backed up and said, "I sure am! Won't you come in? I've made some iced tea, would you like a glass?"

"Sure, anything cold on a hot day is welcome."

She whirled around then said over her shoulder, "Have a seat, I'll be right back."

Roger smiled. "Sure, thanks."

Roger stepped inside and watched as she wheeled herself away. She wore her hair short, but he was sure the waves were natural and the color was a rich honey. He sighed, too bad she was already spoken for he could probably live with a wheelchair running around his home if the contents were something like this. All at once, his bachelorhood wasn't so appealing.

He hurriedly took the seat she'd motioned him to just as she set a tray on her lap in the kitchen and wheeled herself a little more sedately back into the sitting room. "So you were practicing. Was that piece for your concert?"

She came, still with her smile in place and handed him a glass, then set the tray from her lap on the chair close by and sighed. "Yes, it's my focal piece. I'll... wait, I'll get my list, they're in the order I want them."

She came back from the kitchen table and handed him a piece of paper. He looked at it, but he wasn't much into classical music so the names and composers meant nothing. When he said nothing, she said, "Ramon suggested this concert be about an hour and a half, I'd say it'll be about ninety minutes with a fifteen minute intermission, this piece'd follow the intermission."

He didn't want to put a wet blanket on the woman's efforts, so he said, as kindly as he could, "Who will you be catering to?"

"A cross segment. I hope to interest everyone. My students in Philly were children."

Roger cleared his throat, still looking at the paper and read through her list of selections, wondering how he could diplomatically say what was on his mind. "Ms Sandy, most of what the people here in town listen to is Bluegrass, Jazz and Country. You don't have anything like that."

She smiled, knowing what he wasn't saying. "I know that, Mr. Clemens, I'm hoping they will look at this as a cultural stimulation."

"Have you done any advertising?"

She sighed, "No, I already have signs up in both stores for my availability to teach piano, I didn't think it'd be too appropriate to put another ad up beside them for something else I'm doing. Isabel, Ted and Alex have been telling people in town and Isabel's told the whole church in Blairsville about the concert. Besides, if the house isn't full it's okay, I'm nervous enough about it without having to play in front of a crowd."

Roger shook his head and looked her in the eye. "From the few minutes on your porch waiting for a pause when you'd hear me knock, there's no need to be nervous, what I heard was fantastic!" He smiled. "I'm not one to go for classical music much and I was duly impressed."

Sandy smiled. "Thanks." She looked at the list in Roger's hand and said, "If you want to make a by-fold, I could make a charcoal that you could copy onto the front."

"You draw, too?" he gasped.

"Yes, I started painting and drawing about the same time as I took piano lessons."

"You make your drawing. When should I come by for it?"

"I could have it ready any time tomorrow."

"Great! I'll come by in the afternoon. I'll make an announcement in church on Sunday about the concert. Do you go to church?"

"Yes, I've been going with Isabel to a church in Blairsville."

He grinned at her. "You could come to ours."

"Isabel says she won't darken your door. Why is that?"

Roger lost the smile on his face, this woman pulled no punches! He cleared his throat and said, "I think Isabel's too staid in her ways. She doesn't like our contemporary music or our fifteen minute talks."

Without any malice, Sandy grew serious, as she said, "Yes, I have a problem with contemporary music that calls itself 'Christian.' To me it seems you're only putting a few trite Christian words, phrases and clichés to sound that was meant to be played in secular auditoriums. If your 'talks' don't include anything about the fact that Jesus, God's Son, came to die and shed His blood so that lost mankind can be saved and go to heaven, then your speaking is totally in vain, Mr. Clemens. I don't mean to be hateful, but that's what church is for, to equip the saints to go out and be salt and light in their community and to bring sinners to the Savior. The church Isabel's been taking me to does that."

"Whew! Ms. Bernard, you've said quite a mouthful!"

She nodded. "Yes, perhaps I have."

She smiled and picked up her tea for a sip. "I'll get that charcoal done so you can have it tomorrow afternoon, Mr. Clemens."

"That'll be good."

Knowing they didn't have anything else to discuss, Roger put his empty glass on the tray and stood up. With a smile, he held his hand out again to shake hers and said, "Thanks, Ms. Bernard, I'll see what I can do about getting the inside of the program to look like something and bring it by when I come for your picture."

"That'll be great! Thanks. Not that I'm excited about giving a concert, but the program might as well look as professional as possible."

"I don't know if you've seen the church, but by Friday I guarantee there'll be a ramp so that you can get yourself inside."

Sandy took his hand and said, "Thanks, Roger, I'll truly appreciate that." *Daddy's not here to carry me inside.*

Roger dropped Sandy's hand and picked up the paper she'd given him. From the door, he said, "I'll see you tomorrow afternoon."

"Could you make it around five o'clock? It's supposed to be quite nice, I may be out painting some of the scenery most of the day."

"Sure! That'll work out great."

She smiled. "I'll see you then."

She watched him through the window as he went to his Jeep. She shook her head and knew why Isabel didn't have anything to do with his church. She'd not been impressed with his spirituality, he never commented on what she'd said should be played or preached in church. If his talks were similar to Reader's Digest articles, then he probably didn't have the real thing in his own heart. She felt sorry for the people who went to church in his building they weren't being fed from the Word, only getting their ears tickled with non-substantial words. Life was too short to waste on non-substantial anything. Eternity was a long time to spend someplace where God wasn't - in Hell.

Ramon and Duncan were about to finish up their discussion when Ramon saw movement on his parking lot. Hoping, but knowing there was no reason for her to come, his heart dropped when he saw the Jag pull to a stop. It bounced, for some reason she wasn't happy, she'd jammed on the brakes. He sighed she was just what he didn't need on a Friday afternoon. Duncan also looked out the window to see a very fashionably dressed woman step from the car. He cleared his throat, knowing how he was dressed, and said, "You seem to have an affinity for women. That one looks like a fashion plate."

Ramon sighed, "She happens to be my mom. I wish her husband would take her to the uttermost parts of the world!"

Duncan was chuckling as the door opened. "Ramon! I found you here!"

"Yes, Mom, what is it you want now?"

"Well, I…" She looked around the room, only then noticing that there was someone else in the room. "I interrupted something."

"Yes, you did. However, since you're here, meet my new associate, Duncan Roads. He'll be going on the hike tomorrow, possibly some more before the end of the season and working with me starting in the spring. Duncan, my mom, Millie Casbah."

Duncan was on his feet with his hand out. "Good to meet you, Ms. Casbah."

Millie allowed Duncan to touch the tips of her fingers then pulled her hand back. "Ramon needs help in this venture. He's never home, why, nobody'd marry him!"

Ramon scowled. "Mom, who said anything about getting married?"

Millie immediately covered her mouth like a school girl and giggled. From behind her hand, she said, "I thought you knew I want some grandchildren and you know you're the only one who can give them to me."

"Yeah, I guess that's true. What was it you wanted?"

Millie looked around the room again. "Where's the cripple?"

Duncan gasped, but Ramon was across the room in an instant and in her face, his dark eyes stony like ice chips. He grabbed her arm in a vice-like grip and took a step toward the open door. He nearly yelled, "Mom, get out! No one talks about Sandy like that and gets away with it. You're not welcome here!"

Cajoling, Millie sliced her other hand through the air, dismissing his words and said, "Come on, you know that's how you think of her!"

Duncan could see Ramon had balled his free hand into a fist. It was all he could do not to plant it somewhere on his mom. "No, it's not, Mom. Most of the time I don't think of her chair. She is so full of life that she makes you forget about it."

Obviously, Millie wasn't listening she was looking around the room, her eyes stopped on the paintings of the panorama. "Where did you get these awesome paintings?"

"Sandy painted them and brought them by. We're both hoping that someone will purchase them, one or all of them."

"That…" Millie cleared her throat, knowing Ramon didn't want to hear the word she had on the tip of her tongue. Ramon obviously knew the word she was about to say, because his hand tightened painfully on her arm. "That woman who's your receptionist painted them?"

"Yes, *Sandy* did."

Millie swallowed. "Umm, would she paint me something? You know I have that spot over the mantel I could hang a painting."

Ramon forced Millie to take another step outside and said, "Mom, I don't know. When was the last time I was in your house? I can't remember the time. If you want her to paint you a picture you'd have to come talk with her. I know you can't go to her cabin, Isabel threw you off her property."

Millie waved her hand, dismissing his words. "She wasn't serious! I can go there. I mean, how *Christian* is that?" she sneered.

Ramon shook his head, still in Millie's face and walking her backward toward the door. "No, you can't. She told me she threw you out and told you never to come back. The way I heard it straight from her, she was dead serious. Isabel doesn't make idle speeches. So, you were telling me what you came here for."

"I was? I don't remember now. Oh, I remember. Alex told me your receptionist is giving a concert next week!"

"Yes, she is. She's playing at the church next Friday evening. She's hoping some people will ask her to give lessons once they hear her."

Millie snorted. "She can't play worth anything! How can she play piano?"

Ramon wanted to smack her mouth instead he tightened his hand on her arm so much he was sure his fingerprints would leave a bruise. Still in her face, he said, "She does, I've heard and watched her. She's a pro. I'm the MC."

Barely inside the door and still moving, because Ramon still propelled her, Millie threw her head back and laughed. "You? You get up in front of people and introduce something? I have visions of that! You couldn't even get up in front of your class in seventh grade and give a five minute speech without stuttering."

"I'm a bit older now, Mom. I'm pretty sure I can do it without stuttering."

"I'll have to come see. Since you have company, I won't stay."

Ramon kept hold of Millie, swung her around so he could reach the door handle. He turned it and nearly flung her out. "That'll be good, Mom. I'll see you some other time."

After Ramon closed the door, Duncan said, "You and your mom don't see eye to eye."

"What gave you your first clue?" Ramon asked, dryly.

Duncan chuckled. "Umm, the hair?"

Just to prove her son wrong, even though he wasn't going to be there, Millie turned her car toward Isabel's cabins. She smiled, knowing the woman only made idle threats she called herself a 'Christian.' Nobody who claimed that title would do something like throw her off the property! Why, that kind of action was unchristian! Millie drove confidently onto Isabel's parking lot, tires crunching on the gravel. She stopped on the far side of Sandy's van, expecting that Isabel wouldn't see her. However, Millie had only stepped out of the car and taken one step toward Sandy's cabin before Isabel came rushing down her steps.

With purpose in her steps, for being an elderly woman, she hurried across the gravel toward her and said, "Millie Casbah, I told you not to come on this property again! Get back in your car and get off my place. Maybe you can act like you do anywhere else and get away with it, but you can't here, now turn around and get out!"

Millie stopped, taken aback by Isabel's vehemence, but didn't turn back toward her car; she was determined to make a liar out of the old woman. Casually, she said, "Isabel, I want to ask that woman to paint me a picture. I saw those she's hung in Ramon's office. He said I had to ask her, so I'm here."

Still advancing toward the detestable woman, Isabel said, "I don't care! I told you to leave the other day and not come back! I still mean it. If you want to talk to Sandy, you'll have to call her or go when she's at Ramon's."

Taking a step backwards, Millie finally realized Isabel was serious, so she asked, "You'd really throw me off your property? How Christian is that?"

Isabel's eyes narrowed as she glared at the other woman. "How Christian were you when you called Sandy those awful names?"

Millie almost laughed. "But you don't consider me a Christian! Why should I act like one just for you?"

"Because you were obnoxious and totally rude to Sandy. I won't have it on my property. Get in your car and don't ever come back! Do I make myself clear?"

"Yes, very clear!" Millie finally realized that Isabel was totally serious. She'd been walking toward her with each word and Millie found herself right beside her car. "Thanks for nothin'," she said.

Millie was angry. People in town didn't treat her like dirt! She pulled the stick into reverse and gunned the car. Only seconds later, she heard a loud thud at the back of her car, felt a sharp pain in her neck and as she put her hand to the back of her neck, she looked into the rearview mirror and discovered to her horror that a tree stood where she'd last seen her trunk. While she still watched, the glass in the back window began sending little lines out from the bottom and soon fell onto the back seat.

"Oh, my!" she whimpered.

Sandy had looked out the window after finishing her practicing. She saw the two women talking and Isabel walking Millie backwards to her car. When she heard the engine race, she knew that Millie was very angry. When she saw the car hit the tree, she was glad the woman hadn't put the stick into drive. There wouldn't have been much left of her van if she'd driven ahead with the same amount of force.

"Goodness! I hope she's not hurt!" Sandy murmured.

Isabel had gone back into her house and didn't seem interested enough to come back out. Sandy, however, opened her door and moved quickly down the walk toward the wrecked car. She couldn't go to the woman, there wasn't sidewalk in that direction, not even gravel, it stopped where the parking lot stopped she couldn't go on grass and dirt, so she sat at the end of her walk and waited until Millie turned off the ignition.

"Could I call someone for you, Mrs. Casbah?" she asked kindly. "I'll call a wrecker."

"Yes," she snapped. "Call the First Bank in Blairsville and ask for Derek Casbah. Tell him I had an accident and he needs to send a tow truck to get me out."

Sandy smiled at the angry woman. "I'll do that, Mrs. Casbah. Should I call an ambulance? I see you're holding your neck. Did you get a whiplash?"

"Probably, but don't call the ambulance, just tell my husband to come for me."

"I will, Mrs. Casbah." Millie didn't say so much as 'thank you'.

Sandy was gone for several minutes and Millie sat in her car. She put her head gingerly on the back of her seat and closed her eyes. When Sandy wheeled back down the walk, Millie pulled herself from the wreck and snapped, "What did you find out?"

"It's all taken care of, Mrs. Casbah. A wrecker is on its way and so's your husband. They'll both be here about the same time, I imagine."

Millie looked at the young woman and asked, "Why are you so kind to me when I've done nothing but be rude and unkind to you?"

Without any hesitation, Sandy said, "Mrs. Casbah, the Book I highly treasure, called the Bible, says, 'Love your enemies and pray for those who persecute you.' (Matt. 5:44) The Lord Himself said those words I must do as He says." She looked at the space between her and where Millie sat in her car and said, "I'm sorry I can't come on the gravel. Do you feel faint? Does your neck hurt, should you lie down?"

Her conscience pricking her, Millie turned her head away from Sandy and snapped, "No, I'll be fine here! You don't need to mess with me I'll be fine here until Derek comes. Go on back in your house."

Ignoring Millie's curt words, Sandy said, "You probably need to lie down. Can you put the seat back and rest your neck against the headrest?"

"I'll do that!" she nearly yelled.

"Here comes a wrecker and a car. Probably the one's your husband."

ELEVEN

"Yes, go on back inside!" She might be feeling badly, but she didn't want her husband to see the woman she'd been mistreating.

Derek stopped on the far side of Sandy's van, while the wrecker backed up to Millie's car. The driver left his wrecker to hook up the wrecked car, but Derek left his car and saw Sandy first. He looked at her and came to her then he said, "Do you know what happened?"

"I guess you must be Mr. Casbah, I'm Sandy Bernard." She smiled at the man and continued, "Mrs. Casbah and Isabel talked here on the gravel and Isabel walked Mrs. Casbah to her car. When she got in, she must have been angry she gunned her car backwards into the tree. I don't know what they said, I was inside."

The man nodded and smiled at the young woman, then held out his hand. "I'm Derek Casbah. You were the one to call."

"Yes, thank you for coming so quickly and getting the wrecker here so soon. Mrs. Casbah's been holding her neck I presume she has a whiplash."

Derek nodded. "Probably so. I'll take her back to the doctor's office so he can check her out. Thanks for calling me."

Still smiling, Sandy said, "Your welcome. I hope the doctor doesn't find anything seriously wrong."

"Thanks, I'll take care of it," he said.

Derek mumbled something else under his breath. Sandy wasn't sure, but she thought he said something about being more concerned about the cost of getting the car fixed than about what could be wrong with his wife. As Derek walked toward the wreckage and his wife, she shook her head and headed back to her porch. She knew how much her daddy adored her mom she couldn't imagine him speaking about her like Mr. Casbah did about his wife.

Only minutes after she was inside, her phone rang and Isabel said, "What's going on out there? How come there's a wrecker?"

"You couldn't see what happened because of my van, but Mrs. Casbah put her car in reverse and smashed into the tree. Her trunk is smashed to the back window and it shattered a minute later. She's been holding her neck ever since, even when I asked her whom I should call. I called her husband and he called the wrecker and came himself. He's out there with her."

"I feel sorry for the man being saddled with her!" Isabel sighed, "I know that isn't very Christian, but she is so obnoxious!"

"She wasn't too polite to me when I asked who I should call."

"Mmm, I'm not surprised."

Soon all was quiet out on the parking lot and Sandy pulled out a piece of art paper and folded it in half. She didn't know how big a piece of paper Roger would use for the program, but she would make it small enough to put on a folded piece of typing paper. She sat for several minutes contemplating what she wanted to portray.

She had just put down the charcoal, satisfied with her work when her phone rang again. She sighed, wishing she'd gotten that answering machine. She wheeled herself toward the phone then picked it up on the third ring again. "Hello?"

"How are you, Dear?"

"Hi, Mom, I'm fine. How's everything there?"

"You're coming home soon, aren't you?"

"No, Mom, my job for Ramon isn't over for another two months. I'm giving a concert next Friday expecting to get some students as a result. I've hung some paintings in a gallery and I have a few ready to ship off to the library in Philly. The scenes around here are awesome and there are so many places to go to paint. I'll be busy for a lifetime, so no I'm not coming home any time soon. Like I said, I'll probably get a chance to get away at Christmas."

"That man you're working for, he's being good to you?"

"What do you mean, Mom?"

"He's not mistreating you?"

"No, of course not! Why?"

"I wondered. He's not proposed marriage to you, has he?"

"Mom, no. Why?"

"Well, you can't marry him!"

"I can't? Why?"

"Well, because… just because."

"You're not making sense, Mom. He's a good man, but there's no need to worry. He'd have to become a Christian before I'd even consider a proposal of marriage."

"Good, good, I was worried about that, of course."

Sandy was sure that wasn't the real reason, but didn't push. "It's good to talk to you, Mom. Good to hear a familiar voice. I'm glad everyone's well. Keep 'em healthy. Love you!"

"Yes, yes. We'll see you sometime, Dear." Sandy hung up and Colleen's eyes filled with tears as she slowly replaced the receiver. Her baby didn't need her any more.

After Roger left Sandy's cabin, he went to Blairsville to the lumberyard. He walked inside, but stopped at a display rack with several colorful booklets in the slots. One of them caught his eye, the title was, 'Decks, Patios and Ramps Made Easy for Beginners.' "Beginner, that's me for sure!" He grumbled. He pulled the booklet from the rack and checked the contents, then turned to a page near the back that displayed only ramps. He sighed; even the most simple one looked to be beyond his knowledge of carpentry. He wasn't at all sure he'd be able to read these plans and where would he get the money for all that wood?

A salesman came over and asked, "Need some help, Sir?"

Giving the man his usual grin, Roger said, "I'm the preacher at the church in Vansville. Next Friday we're to have a concert put on by a lady in a wheelchair. The church has never had a ramp, there hasn't been a need, but there are five steps to get from the sidewalk to the front door, the back door is the same." Roger made a face and said, "I'm thinking I need a ramp desperately and in a hurry. How's the best way to get one cheap and fast?"

"Hmm, you do have a problem, don't you?"

Roger nodded and brushed his hand through his hair. "Yeah, especially when I'm not too sure which end is the business end of a hammer."

The man stood looking over Roger's shoulder at the pictures, then motioned with his head, "Come on over to this table and let's talk about it."

A half hour later, the two men stood and shook hands. Roger walked out of the place with his booklet and a receipt in hand. On the way to his Jeep he took another look at the receipt and shook his head. He wished he'd insisted that there be admission charged for the concert, that every adult who came paid ten dollars and each child's ticket was five. He shook his head, even if every seat was taken, that amount of money wouldn't cover the thousand dollar cost for the order that would be delivered to the church tomorrow. Even if he got all the men who came to church and all the men whose wives came, he still wasn't sure he'd get the job done. His expertise on carpentry was non-existent and he wasn't too sure about anyone else in town. Ramon was good with a hammer, but he'd be gone all week with his hikers.

He slammed the door to his Jeep and put the key in the ignition. Somehow he'd find the money thank goodness he'd gotten a discount because it was for a church. He'd get the ramp built before Friday night. People were already advertising the concert and he was sure that for the guest musician it would be the highest insult for a bunch of men to have to carry her up the steps into the building for her own concert. He grinned and his mood lightened immediately, actually, he wouldn't mind carrying Ms Sandy Bernard anywhere the lovely lady would want to go. He knew Ramon had something for her, but did he know just what he'd gotten? Well, for goodness sake! He was 'a man of the cloth' – *Clemens, behave yourself!*

Not long after the wrecker left Isabel's parking lot with Millie's car and Derek left with Millie, a white truck with bold letters on all sides squealed around the corner from the road onto Isabel's parking lot. His truck was still jerking when he jumped out with a huge box and headed for the office. He bounded up the steps and banged on the door, balancing the box in one arm, but turned to look at the brand new blue van parked across the way.

Isabel came to the door and opened it with a scowl. "Yes?"

The man looked at his clipboard and asked, "Sandra Bernard?"

Isabel shook her head. "No, she's in that cabin over where the blue van is parked."

"Okay, thanks, Ma'am." In two steps the man was off Isabel's porch and with long strides went across the gravel behind the van and up to Sandy's porch. Again he knocked loudly, then stepped back and waited.

Sandy was painting on her last canvas. She laid her brush down on the easel, but still held her pallet, as she wheeled herself to the door. She had the advantage of seeing the big truck through her front window, so she knew who was knocking. She pulled the door open and smiled at the man. "Hi, you have a package for me?"

"Yes, Ma'am, you're Sandra Bernard?" When she nodded, he said, "I need your signature on this form."

"Why don't you bring that box in here and I'll sign your paper."

Sandy backed up and laid her pallet on the coffee table, then reached for the man's clipboard. The man held it out to her then after Sandy took it, he let the box slide down his arm to the floor. Sandy signed her name, then held the clipboard out and said, "Here you go! Would you like a glass of iced tea before you go?"

The man shook his head. "No, Ma'am, I'm running late, thanks, though."

"Sure! You have a good weekend."

The man grinned back at her and said, "I intend to, thanks."

Sandy closed the door and stared at the huge box. It couldn't be heavy, the man had carried it in one arm, but unless she could push it with her footrest, she knew she'd never get it in the closet. Knowing that Ramon was busy with Duncan, meant she wouldn't call him to put a box away. Isabel was an old lady, she didn't want to tax her so she leaned over and pushed the box until it was in her traveling lane. It took quite a while to move the box from the door to the closet then she had a problem reaching the door knob to push it open. Finally she had the box in her closet and opened it. As she expected, inside were several sizes of canvases. She smiled, glad they'd come. If they hadn't come today, they wouldn't have come for three days. If possible, she liked to do some art work each day, just to keep her hand in it. If the canvases hadn't come today, she'd have had to restrict herself to doing charcoals on typing paper.

As she sat there looking at them, a thought crossed her mind. Her smile grew larger and her eyes sparkled. "Yes! I'll do it!" she exclaimed.

After she ate, she called Roger to come for his picture, then Isabel and said, "Hi, it's me. That box was full of canvases. I've decided to go on a painting excursion this weekend, since I have three days off from Ramon's."

"Missy, where will you go?"

"Isabel, I don't know, around on some of the back roads so I can paint some of God's simply fantastic scenes. I wanted to tell you so you wouldn't worry when my van's gone."

"Okay, Missy, you have a great time!"

"Don't you worry about that! I'm sure I will."

Saturday morning dawned sunny and warm. Ramon was up with the sun and fixed a pot of coffee. Last night after Duncan had left, he'd set all the food he'd bought for this hike by the door in the office, except for a bit of fresh fruit that he would get out of his fridge in the morning. The fruit, some zip bags filled with the right amount of coffee for his percolator and several boxes of breakfast bars were the only exceptions to the packages of dried food that would be reconstituted with the water from the creeks they'd camp beside each night. When the hikers came, he'd distribute everything among them for their backpacks.

Duncan should arrive soon for breakfast and a last minute look at the map. They'd talked at length about the use of a computer yesterday and Ramon was convinced he must get one. Charting the trips and viewing the terrain from the internet seemed like a good way to expand their hikes to other parts of the area. It would work well with two guides.

This year Ramon had only done a few variations in his trips. To his surprise, the pictures on the internet showed several trails he wasn't aware of. It wet his appetite to find them and check them out even this year. He and Duncan were seasoned hikers and backpackers without any family strings they could do the exploring after the season was over for paid trips. He was excited to see some of these places. In years past, when he hadn't been so busy, he'd hiked in some of the areas, but never taken a group.

A car door slammed and Ramon saw the SUV parked on the lot. He went to the door and opened it, waiting for Duncan to come. The big man was dressed as he had been the day before, in jeans and a short sleeved plaid shirt and hiking boots. His hair was pulled into a ponytail and hung down his back. He pulled his backpack from the back and leaned it up against his vehicle then he pulled a much smaller object out and holding the handle, came toward Ramon.

The smile split his facial hair and his eyes twinkled, as he said, "Hi, Ramon! I'm hungry as a bear and I smell coffee."

Ramon chuckled. "I fixed some waffles and of course the coffee. Come on in, I've spread the map on the table along with our places."

"Great! I brought my laptop so I can locate the area. I slept well, but woke up early."

Duncan sat down and Ramon filled a bowl with scrambled eggs. As he pulled out his chair, he sighed, "You'll never guess what Mom did! She left here and went directly to the cabins she wasn't allowed to visit. Just as I warned her, the lady threw her off the property, it made Mom mad and she wrecked her car."

"I'm sorry to hear that. Was she hurt badly?"

Ramon shook his head. "Just whiplash, she backed into a tree and wound her trunk around it. She'll live, of course, but her car won't. Derek had it towed into Blairsville, but even if he had it fixed, Mom wouldn't drive it again. He told me he might leave her without a car for a while. I can't say as I blame him."

"That'll put a damper on her for a bit."

"Believe me, not long enough. She calls or comes by each week, at least once."

They both flopped a huge waffle on their plates, lathered some soft butter across the surface and then drowned it in a sea of sweet syrup. Duncan did something Ramon had never seen a man do, he opened his shirt and tucked his beard inside it, then cut a big square of waffle and stuffed it in his mouth, then as the rich sweetness registered on his tongue he groaned his satisfaction. "Delicious!"

After they'd been eating for a while, Duncan said, "Is Sandy related to you?"

"No, why do you ask?"

Duncan shrugged. "You hold a torch for her I thought perhaps she was your sister."

Ramon wiped his mouth and took a long slug from his coffee mug, before he said, "No, she's from Philadelphia and came last month for an interview. I hired her and she's done a fantastic job with my office." Ramon shook his head. "I almost didn't hire her, since there's so little left of the season, but she's been fantastic!"

"But you… I don't know… Is she your girlfriend?"

Ramon's dark skin didn't show a blush too much, and he couldn't remember the last time he'd been embarrassed or self-conscious, especially with another man, but he could feel his neck and cheeks getting hot. Had his feelings for the beautiful young woman showed that much? He wiped his mouth on his napkin, stalling. He finally said, "We aren't dating, I took her for an afternoon to see some of the area, since she's an artist and not from here. She's fixed me a couple of meals, both times after I'd returned in the rain from a hike. I haven't thought of her as my girlfriend." *Liar*, the little voice said from his shoulder. *You know you'd take her to your bed in a minute if you could, old man.*

Not knowing Ramon's thoughts, Duncan speared the last mouthful of waffle and stuffed it in his mouth, chewed and swallowed, then took a long, thoughtful draw on his coffee, then turned to Ramon with a scowl of his own. "But she's in a wheelchair, she can't walk. From what you've said, she never has and she never will."

Not understanding where Duncan was going with this, he asked, "Why is that a problem for you? She does a fantastic job with everything she does. Her paintings are first rate," He pointed down the hall to the room where the paintings hung that Duncan had helped him hang. "and she plays like a concert pianist. The meals she's cooked were fit for a king. She's so happy and vivacious, no one who really knows her thinks about her chair. I hardly notice and I get much more defensive with people who down-grade her because of her chair than she does."

Duncan sighed and leaned back in his chair, holding his mug. "I guess my problem is that I've always been such an outdoors man and been in perfect health all my life that to see someone who's not it pricks my conscience or something. I, umm, sort of didn't treat her very well by not shaking her hand that she offered me."

"I noticed, but did she make you feel badly because you didn't?"

"No, that's what makes me feel even worse."

Ramon smiled at him. "It's okay, it's allowed once."

Duncan nodded. "I'll remember that."

By the time the four hikers arrived, Duncan and Ramon had outlined their route on the map and had it entered into Duncan's computer. They both had their share of the food stored in their backpacks and were ready for the hikers. The sun was out bright and strong and Ramon had a smile on his face as he saw the four vehicles drive up. One of them parked in the spot where a light blue van usually parked and Ramon was pushing his chair back to go tell the driver to move, when it hit him, Sandy wouldn't be here at all during the time they'd be gone. He slumped back and let out a sigh. That also meant he wouldn't see the lovely lady for three long days. Man, did he have it bad or what?

The four men entered Ramon's office and both men inside stood up. "Hi, guys!" Ramon had his hand out, wanting to greet his friends. "It's great to see you! Meet my new associate, Duncan Roads. He's going with us and then he's coming on board as a guide. He'll be starting officially next spring."

"Great to meet you, Duncan," one man said.

The four men had their hands out as Duncan went around and shook each of their hands. Grinning, he said, "Howdy, fellas, I'm pleased to meet you. Looks like we've really lucked out on the weather for this weekend."

After the introductions, one of the men asked, "So where do we go from here? Do we walk or drive to the trail head?"

Nodding at the pile by the door, Ramon said, "You guys'll need to divide up those food stuffs into your backpacks, then we'll get into Duncan's SUV and drive down the road a ways. We'll park on the dirt road then walk to the trail head. It shouldn't take but about a half hour to reach the place."

"Okay, let's be about it! I came here to hike, not jaw."

As the men stuffed the food into their packs, one asked, "Hey, Ramon, who's the female who answered your phone when I called to confirm?" He winked at Ramon. "Your live-in?"

"She's Sandy Bernard, my receptionist."

The young man scowled then picked up another package for his pack. "When did you decide you needed one of those?"

"When too many people complained they didn't like talking to a mailbox all the time, so of course, I lost some business that way, because who knows how many of those there are. I've had trips almost back to back all season, so I'm rarely here. She's been running the office quite efficiently for about a month. She's even done a little expanding for me, too."

"She'll stay through the winter?"

"She's moved here permanently, so she says. I don't know if she'll be available next spring, we haven't talked about it."

Ramon looked around at the backpacks that were full and the empty space beside his door. "I guess we're ready to move, aren't we?"

"Appears so. Lead on, man!"

Just as they were heading out the door, one of the hikers looked up at the paintings on the wall and exclaimed, "Ramon! Isn't that the panorama from that lookout down the road a ways? Those pictures are awesome! Where did you get them?"

His hand on the door knob, Ramon grinned and said, "It sure is, that's exactly where they're from. I was hoping somebody'd notice."

"Wow! Where did you get **paintings** of it?"

"My receptionist, Sandy, painted them after I took her there one afternoon not long ago. Two she painted from memory, the other two from photos."

The hiker shook his head. "Wow! They are something awesome!"

Ramon grinned. "They're for sale if anybody's interested."

"Ah, so you have a gallery now!"

"Yup! Right up town!"

When they reached the parking lot, Duncan opened the back of his SUV and loaded all the backpacks and one man tents inside. After everyone climbed in, the four hikers in the back two seats and Ramon in the front passenger seat, Duncan said, "Okay, Ramon, tell me the way."

"Turn left from my parking lot and head out of town."

Anxious to get on the trail, Duncan said, "We're on it, man!"

Sandy was up early, she'd gone to bed early, right after getting supplies together for three days of meals, some extra clothes and half the canvases that came in the huge box and of course, all her paints and easel. She was excited and so happy that she'd thought to go on this excursion. She dressed comfortably, ate her breakfast and started taking her things to the van. She was loaded, had her back seat down and was in the driver's seat before she saw any movement in Isabel's house, not that she'd expected the lady to watch her or to come out and speak to her. They were neighbors who acted like any others.

Ramon had several maps of the area in his office and she'd taken one of each different one when she'd first arrived in town, perhaps it was a vicarious wish to learn where he went. None of them used Vansville as a focal point, but it wasn't hard to locate where it was, since it was in the center of the trails leading into the hills and mountains.

She drove away from the cabins and soon was in the country. She followed the road Ramon had taken her on for their afternoon outing a week or so ago, then turned off of it onto a dirt road that was beyond where they'd stopped for lunch. Not far off the main road, she found a pull off, so she stopped and parked. Her smile was brilliant as she lowered herself to the ground.

It hadn't rained for almost a week, so the dirt was dry and well packed, so Sandy set off to do some exploring. Where she was parked was in some trees, but she was sure that around the corner she'd find something sensational to paint. That corner came quickly and she was rewarded with a view that made her gasp.

She hurried back to her van, pulled out her easel and a canvas, her brushes and her case of paints. Since she couldn't see her van from around the corner, she locked it up and set off for her view, which she planned to paint to her heart's content. She'd send some of these paintings to Philly to the library. She knew they'd sell.

The big SUV traveled down the highway for several miles after leaving Vansville. The men were laughing and joking, they didn't know each other well, but they all knew Ramon and that was enough to become quick friends. Ten miles out of town, Ramon told Duncan to turn onto a dirt road, that was a glorified name for a cowpath, two tiretracks wide. The trees were huge and full of leaves, without a trace of fall color. The branches hung over the road, nearly blotting out the sun. They couldn't see any signs of civilization, only the cowpath, trees and sky.

They had made three turns from the road and so couldn't be seen from it when one of the hikers said, "What's reflecting the sun up ahead there?"

Ramon was half turned in his seat so he could easily chat with his friends and he was looking at them over his shoulder. When the man spoke, his head whipped around and he stared, open mouthed at the metal that reflected the sun. Before he could get his mouth closed, Duncan said, "It's a blue van!"

"It sure is!" another man said.

"That's right where I was going to direct you to park," Ramon said, in a very subdued voice. "Besides, that's Sandy's van."

"Sandy's van! What's she doing here?" Duncan asked, incredulous. He looked at his new friend. "You didn't tell her to come here, did you?"

Ramon scowled at his associate. "Of course not! I had no idea she planned to come! She's probably painting the scene we'll see up ahead." Duncan had slowed to a crawl, but Ramon motioned him on by the van and said, "There's another pull off up a bit farther, we'll go on to it and park there."

"I won't run her down, will I?"

Ramon shrugged and grinned. "You could be a little careful and watch the road some."

"Yeah, right!" Duncan grumbled.

The men in the backseats didn't know Sandy, other than what one of them had asked Ramon about her pictures. They didn't know she was in a wheelchair. All four of them threw their heads back and howled with laughter until Duncan turned the corner and all six of them saw the easel and the chair holding the artist. Then the little space inside the SUV became deathly quiet, as the six men looked out the windshield.

Sandy had moved off the dirt trail enough that Duncan could pull by her, if he moved as far to the other side as he could. As she had with Ramon at the pull off on the highway from Blairsville, she totally ignored the big vehicle as he inched by her. Ramon's heart rate tripled the minute he saw her. The two men on the far side of the van strained across the other two so they could see Sandy's painting. None of them looked at the view she was painting.

One of the men asked, "That's your receptionist?"

Ramon had to lick his lips. "Yes, that's Sandy. I didn't know she'd come here to paint!"

"You haven't distracted her at all by pulling by her, Duncan. I should think she'd be afraid way back in here off the road where no one can see her. We could be some criminal intent on hiding out and doing some damage or hurting people in the area."

Ramon remembered how she was at the pull off and said, "She's concentrating on the lighting. She doesn't let anything distract her while she's painting if she can help it. She was that way when I saw her at the pull-off near Blairsville."

Duncan swallowed as he pulled back onto the dirt trails several feet ahead of her. "So where do I park this thing, Man?"

"Up around this next curve is another pull off, we'll take that."

When Duncan found the pull off, he nosed his SUV into the place, pulling the hood almost into the branches of the trees. The men opened the doors and scrambled out. They heard nothing. Their vehicle had made enough noise that it had scared the birds into silence and they were far enough from the road that no traffic noises came to them. Sandy, of course, was several car lengths away and she made no noise while she painted. It could be the middle of nowhere.

Ramon's greatest desire was to go back up the road to see Sandy and see what she was painting. He knew it'd be awesome. However, he stood at the back of the SUV, waiting for Duncan to pull out his backpack. As Duncan hauled out his pack, he said to Ramon, "You gonna go see her... see what she's painting?"

"And be a distraction? When I stopped that day on the pull-off near Blairsville, she wouldn't look at me, but kept on painting. She'd probably be just as happy if we don't show."

Duncan shrugged. "Whatever you say."

Not knowing what Duncan sensed about Ramon and Sandy, one hiker said, "Why? An artist is an artist, we got hiking to do and only three days to do it in, let's get on a trail!"

"My thoughts exactly!" another young man added.

Duncan shrugged and looked at his watch. "I guess you have a point. I've never seen a real artist in action, that's all."

Ramon shouldered his pack and said, "We go almost back to where she is."

Of course, Sandy had heard the big vehicle coming before she saw it. It had been very quiet ever since she'd set up her easel, no birds even chirped. She was surprised that she'd found the exact road that Ramon planned to use as his parking place for this hike. When they'd come out that afternoon, he'd turned around after they ate lunch and gone another way, so she didn't know the exact location where he started off.

However, she wouldn't let him or anyone else distract her. The sun sparkled off one rock on the far view and she knew it wouldn't stay bright very long. She was well aware of the van as it went by, but she didn't acknowledge it. She wondered briefly if Ramon or any of the men would come back to see her. She dabbed her brush into another color, mixed it with the color already on her pallet and went on painting. If they came back was soon enough to think about it.

Early Saturday morning, Roger pulled out his list of faithful attendees. He looked down the list and made a face. Most were women whose husbands didn't come with them. For the first time, he wondered why that was. He wasn't conceited enough to think they came because of him. When his finger found the first man's name, he dialed and waited through three rings.

A man's sleepy voice answered, "Hullo?"

"Hi, Corky, it's Roger Clemens, did I wake you?"

"I's just layin' here thinkin' I'd better get up. You didn't wake me, I was just dozin' by my wife, you know? What's up, Preacher?"

"Are you busy today?"

"Just honeydo stuff, why?"

"You know about the concert at church Friday night?"

"Yeah..." the man said, tentatively.

"The lady's in a wheelchair. You know what that means?"

There was a pause before the man said, "No, don't rightly think so...."

"It means we need a ramp from the sidewalk to the front door in less than a week. You got time today to help me build it?"

"A ramp! At our church?"

"That's what I'm sayin', Corky."

"You got plans and stuff?"

"I got the plans and the stuff's coming from the lumberyard this morning."

"Sure, I'll help for a while you know them honeydo things don't like to wait much, if you get my drift?"

"Sure, Corky, any time you can give will be appreciated."

Roger made several more calls and received about the same response. By the time he had half a dozen committed, he'd decided to supply drinks and lunch. His meager budget was already strained with normal living expenses, but perhaps his hens would lay a few more eggs and he'd get a few extra bucks for them. Of course he wouldn't starve if he missed a meal or two once in a while.

He poured the last of his coffee into his insulated cup, slapped the cap on it and jumped in his Jeep. He headed down his driveway and looked at the dash clock. The truck with the lumber should be pulling up to the church about the time he arrived. He hoped Ms. Bernard would be impressed with the job when he and his men had it finished. After all, she was the only reason he was doing this. For that matter, she didn't even go to his church, for crying out loud!

It was a simple design, the simplest and the least expensive in the book. It was a good thing most of the men only brought a hammer, probably from the collection of tools they kept for honeydo jobs. Corky had a tool belt that he buckled around his ample waist when he climbed from his truck. Roger ran across the street to the hardware store when it opened to buy his hammer. He couldn't find one at home.

The first thing Corky asked was, "Anyone got a screw gun or a circular saw?"

Roger scowled. "No, we need one? The lumberyard guy didn't mention that."

The other man shrugged. "A deck or ramp goes together with a lot less effort and a lot faster with a screw gun." He grinned. "Fortunately, I have mine here in my toolbox. Did the lumberyard say if they were sending nails or screws?"

Roger frowned. "I'm not sure, Corky. I don't remember if we even talked about anything but the wood."

"Hmm, that would be a problem."

Chuckling, Roger said, "Yes, I guess it would be, wouldn't it? I knew we needed lumber, but I never thought about what to put it together with."

They saw a large truck coming down the road and as it approached the intersection the turn signal came on. The truck turned onto the side street close to the curb so that the back of the truck was close to the very front of the church. The driver and his helper got out and came to the back where the church men had gathered.

"Roger Clemens?"

Roger stepped forward. "That would be me."

Before anyone else spoke, the man with the tool belt asked, "Did you fellas bring nails or screws for this job?"

The driver shook his head. "Have no idea. The yard supervisor had this loaded yesterday while I was delivering another order. He gave me this sheet this morning to get signed when I got here. We're to unload and head on back."

The man shrugged. "I guess we'll find out as we unload."

"Seems so. So, this a good place for you?"

"Yeah," Corky said, "We'll make it work."

The two from the lumberyard turned toward the truck. The older man climbed onto the flatbed and climbed onto the loader, while the younger man unlocked the travel restraints. Soon the man fired up the machine and moved to the front of the truck, then pushed his tongs under a pallet. While he did that, the younger man pulled out some long ramps and laid the far end on the ground. The backup beeper on the loading machine came on and the man turned around to make sure he was headed for those ramps.

While he moved down the ramp, the other man climbed up on the truck and walked around the moving load. He picked up several smaller boxes and brought them to the side of the truck. The church men moved over and each one grabbed a box. When the loader was on the ground, the man took the load to the grass close to the walk and set it down. He went back up the ramp, engaged another smaller pile on another pallet and brought it down to the ground. By this time, all the men had the smaller boxes unloaded and were standing around again.

After the ramp and the loader were back in place, the driver brought his clipboard to Roger for him to sign. The man with the tool belt said, "Wait, a minute. Let's check to see if they brought screws or nails. We'd really rather have screws. If he brought nails, he can take them back. I'll follow him back and make the trade."

The lumber employee shrugged and said, "It's okay by me."

He read the list over Roger's shoulder then breathed a sigh, as he read the last line. "Ahh, they sent screws. Go ahead and sign, Roger."

The truck pulled away, leaving Roger staring at the pile and scratching his head. "Corky," he said, "I sure hope you can make some sense out of this pile of sticks."

"Sure! First off, we need my posthole digger to make holes for the uprights we need to sink along the sides. Have you outlined where you want the ramp?"

Roger scowled and shook his head. "All I know, I picked up this booklet at the lumberyard and got stuff for the cheapest one."

"Hmm, may have a problem. Let's figure it out, put down the stakes and go from there."

Before long, two of the ladies from the church drove up and began to set up a table on the sidewalk close to where the men were working. They put up a beach umbrella and unfolded several chairs under it. When they were all set up, they brought two coolers from the trunk, then set them both in the shade of the table, then one of them went across the street and down a ways to the grocery store and came back with two large bags of ice. They immediately filled one cooler with the ice, but left the other one closed up.

When they finished, one of the ladies called to the men, "Say, guys, we brought iced tea, lemonade and soft drinks. You tell us when you want lunch we brought roast beef sandwiches when you're ready for them."

Roger rushed over to the ladies and exclaimed, "Wow! You're a lifesaver! You ladies are great! Thanks!"

"Hey, no problem. It's still summer and the forecast said it's headed for another scorcher today, so we thought some refreshment was in order."

"I'm much obliged, thanks."

"Hey, it's cool! You're doing this for that Sandy woman aren't you, the one who has the paintings in the store windows?"

"Yes, Sandy Bernard's playing this coming Friday and she's in a wheelchair."

"What's she play?" one of the men called to him.

"She plays piano. Ramon says she hopes for some interest for her lessons from this."

Melvin stood up and looked from the plans booklet to the area they were clearing, then to Roger and asked, "She plays what?"

"The piano, man, she's good, I've heard her."

Shaking his head, he scowled and asked, "How does she play piano if she needs a ramp to get into the building?"

"Beats me!" Roger exclaimed. "All I know is she's in a wheelchair. I heard her from inside when I was on her porch, but she came to the door to let me in."

"I'll be jimswiggled!" the older man exclaimed. "A cripple plays piano, that's the craziest thing I ever heard!"

By the end of the day, after all the drinks and roast beef sandwiches had disappeared and all the volunteer labor had gone home to their honey-do jobs, Roger stood back to survey their day's work. He was a bit disappointed, all they'd done was dig holes, set posts and pour cement around the posts into the holes. Fortunately, the men he'd called knew more about building than he did. They all volunteered to return on Tuesday after work to start connecting the posts with all the lumber that Roger had bought, most of which still sat on the tree plot. They assured him it would be ready by Friday.

He looked at the scattered posts that were held erect and straight by pieces of the lumber that they hadn't used yet. Yorky had made sure the supports they'd cut were cut to the exact length they'd need for the ramp. Several of the posts had four pieces, one for each side. Corky said they couldn't do anything until Tuesday because the cement had to cure. He guessed that meant harden so they could take down the boards. Between now and then he was supposed to come up with a heavy duty seventy-five foot extension cord to hook up inside so Corky could run his screw gun and fasten everything together.

He looked at the pitiful amount of work they'd done and the huge pile of lumber still lying on the grass and mumbled, "Sure, it'll be done before Friday! Corky even said we need to put some kind of sealer on this! How can that dry by Friday?" Discouraged, he climbed back into his Jeep and left for his quiet acres. He grinned maybe he'd have to carry the lovely Ms Bernard into his church after all. He chuckled cynically at his own joke. If anybody had to carry Ms Bernard he was sure he knew who would do it and it wouldn't be him!

TWELVE

Ramon had his tent tied on his pack, so he waited until the others had theirs tied in place. Standing in the right wheel track, he said, "We go back this way to the trailhead."

One man smirked, "You mean back to the artist?"

Ramon didn't rise to the bait. "Remember I told you I'd planned to park where the blue van is parked? That's because right across this road is where we go through the trees to reach the trail." He grinned at his friend. "So, we go back to the artist, yes."

The man shrugged, "Fair enough, let's go!"

Sandy heard their voices and she could tell when they began to move closer to her. She continued to paint, the light was changing and she hadn't gotten the rock to suit her yet. Ramon didn't know how well their voices carried, so when they could see her, he called, "Sandy, we're back here, but we must walk on by to the trailhead."

"That's fine, Ramon, I'm sorry I took your parking place, but hey, there wasn't a sign."

He chuckled and said, "It's no big deal, these guys need to work off some extra steam. They've been giving me a hassle ever since they came. Are you at a stopping place so I could introduce you to these bundles of testosterone?"

Sandy put her brush on the easel ledge and whirled herself around in place. She smiled up at the five handsome men who stood with Ramon and self-consciously, they smiled back at her. If they'd been asked, they'd have had to admit to Duncan's mindset, they were all robust outdoorsmen, but to a man, they were uncomfortable in Sandy's presence. Ramon said, "Sandy, this is Duncan, you met him yesterday. This is Dave, Eric, Rob and Sylvester. Except for Duncan, of course, they've all been hiking with me before."

Sandy still smiled, but said, "I won't shake your hands, fellas I've gotten some paint on my fingers that would get on you. I'm happy to meet you all. Ramon's been looking forward to this hike. I've heard the weather's to be fantastic, so have a great time and don't get hurt. We had that happen not long ago, so be careful."

One man stepped forward and looked at her painting, then looked up beyond at the real thing. "Wow! You're really good!"

She smiled at the young man. "Thanks, Rob, I love to paint and I've been doing it for quite a few years."

"It shows. Ramon said you painted the ones back at his office. I've seen that panorama, except it was a different season when I saw it it looks exactly like what you see out there."

Sandy smiled. "Thanks." She nodded over her shoulder. "I'd better get back to it, the light changes so fast, you know."

Before the men even moved, Sandy whirled her chair around again and picked up her brush. She was slathering paint on the canvas even before the men were out of sight. She was so caught up in what she was doing the men heard her humming before they turned off the road onto the trail. For several minutes, no one said anything. Ramon was anxious to hear what the men had to say, once they were out of Sandy's hearing.

"She's great! That scene was awesome she was painting!"

Ramon nodded. "Yes, that picture and the ones of the panorama don't have anything but scenery in them, but the very first one I saw and bought from her has an eagle in it. It's the most awesome bird I've ever seen painted. I saw it flying there at the turnoff, but on my wall, it looks like he's floating on air."

"She wants to sell those?"

"Yes, she'll sell those four at my office and I'm sure this one'll be for sale, too."

"She's not bitter because she's in that chair?"

"Not that I can see. I've never seen her down she's always cheerful and totally vivacious. Even on rainy days, she's like that."

"Must be a Christian," one man said, softly.

Ramon answered, "Yes, that's what she says. She's told me I ought to be one, too."

Eric said, "It can't hurt you, man!"

It was Sunday. The friends had had a super time together on Saturday and the weather had been perfect for them, the sun bright, the breeze comfortable. They'd sweat a lot in the early September heat, but last evening they'd camped beside a cool, refreshing stream and each of them had taken full advantage of the deep pools that were close to their camp site. They'd covered some rough terrain, but were glad for the challenge, since that's what they came for. Last night had been clear and still, they'd let the fire burn low and only laid out their sleeping bags to sleep. It was a night to remember. The mosquitoes hadn't had the nerve to bother them.

All day Sunday Eric was very quiet as they hiked along. Finally, Rob said to him, "What's with you, man? We're in the great out-of-doors in the most perfect of places. We've all become great buddies. You should be ecstatic with this trip! What gives?"

Eric shrugged. "I know all that, but something's really getting to me."

"Well, spill it, man!"

Eric sat down on a fallen log beside the trail, so the others joined him, two sitting beside him the rest sitting on the ground in front of him. Immediately, they all uncapped their canteens for a long drink. After a long draw from his canteen, Eric capped it and said, "I can't get it all into words, but what I can say is that up to last week I've lived all of my twenty-six years scoffing and shaking my fist at God Almighty. Something happened last week that brought me to my knees and showed me how wrong I was. I became a Christian, a Believer in the One True God, who made heaven and earth and all there is in it, but yet He's interested and listens to me. He loved me enough to send His own beloved Son to an old rugged cross to die to pardon my sins and make me a new person and then in three days he came out of that grave to live again. I still can't fathom all that means."

"You've become a Christian!" Ramon said, in awe, it wasn't a question. "Sandy's talked like that several times since she came."

Eric nodded. "Yes, a week ago yesterday I finally gave in and told God he could have everything, good and bad, but mostly bad, that there was about me. A peace I've never known came over me, but it's overwhelming. Now I'm out here in this wilderness and even though I've hiked in places like this before, it's like it's all new. I don't know, everything I see seems to show me God's work, He's so close I feel like I'm about to burst with it all."

"Ahh, come on, man!" Duncan exclaimed. "Get over it! We got hiking to do, we can't be side tracked by some preacher boy."

"I'm with you!" Sylvester muttered.

His chin in his chest, Eric shook his head and said, "I'm not a preacher boy, Duncan. If you'd known me before, you'd never say that. I've done some things I'm not proud of at all, but I can say truthfully that God's taken it all away because Jesus, His Son, died for me."

The rest of the men looked at each other, but didn't say anything. Finally Eric clamped his canteen onto the strap of his backpack and started down the trail. The others scrambled to their feet and caught up to him. Duncan and the other three men quickly passed him and went back to their carefree tramp through the woods, but Ramon fell back beside Eric and silently walked with him.

It seemed God was pursuing him, too. He'd been confronted several times, some in a very powerful way, this summer, much more than any other year. Of course, there was Sandy she was the most powerful confrontation of them all. He couldn't refute her life, he didn't know many people who were handicapped, but those he did never were as happy as she. There was not any bitterness in her at all. He was sure it was because she was a Christian.

The sun was casting long shadows through the trees when they finally heard a fast moving stream close by. There was a wide grassy area off to one side of the trail and the stream bordered it on the far side. Without saying anything, Duncan unbuckled his backpack from his waist even as he saw the spot a hundred yards in front of them. Again today they'd been hot and sweaty, not from humidity, but hard hiking. In only minutes, all six of the men had shed everything and were dashing into the cold mountain water. Even before they were completely submerged, goose bumps covered their skin.

After letting their bodies dry and dressing again, they pulled out food packages for supper and started the fire. Each of them heated water that they'd purified and fixed their meal. There were a few mosquitoes around this stream, so four of the men set up their tents, but Eric and Ramon only rolled out their sleeping bags close together with their feet close to the fire. For about an hour as the stars came out and the fire died down, the men told some experience they'd had in the past year, but soon, four of the men headed for their tents.

Ramon lay on his sleeping bag with his hands behind his head and gazed at the stars that shone brilliantly, since there were no large cities to throw their lights into the heavens. The day they'd spent had been awesome and he too, had felt an overwhelming Presence close beside him all day. He knew Eric wasn't sleeping yet, he also lay with his hands under his head staring at the brilliant stars. Finally, Ramon said, "Tell me about your experience last week."

Taking a long breath, Eric finally said, "I met this new woman at work. She's the most beautiful woman I've ever seen. I asked her out, wanted to get to know her, but she turned me down flat. After I got my breath back, I asked her why. She said, 'I know from the way you talk and act and the company you keep you aren't a Christian.' I scowled at her and said, 'So?' She shook her head, looked me straight in the eye and said, 'I will not go on one date with anyone who is not a Believer in Jesus who is God's Son and the Savior of mankind.' I just looked at her." He shook his head. "Believe me I'd never in all my life since I discovered women had one turn me down for a reason like that!"

"So she read to you from her Bible?"

"Not right then, we had to get back to work. Besides, it bugged me for several days that she'd turn me down. Another day, I saw her again and she was reading it. I asked her about it and she said, 'Have you ever heard of the Romans Road?' I shrugged and said, 'No, I don't think so, is it here in the country?' She smiled a little, but shook her head."

"What's that?" Ramon asked. "Was it somewhere close by? What could it have to do with reading the Bible?"

Eric scrambled from his bag and rummaged in his backpack. "I'll show you what she showed me. You'll understand then."

Ramon shrugged. "Okay."

As soon as Eric straightened from his pack, Ramon had a flashback to the group he'd taken a week ago. Eric walked back to his seat with a small book and a pinpoint flashlight. He sprawled on his sleeping bag on his stomach and shined the light on the Book. Ramon knew it was a Bible just like the pastor had. Eric held the light and opened the Book toward the back.

"The Romans Road is called that because everything I'm reading is found in the Bible in the book of Romans. The first is 3:23: '...for all have sinned and fall short of the glory of God.' The next is 6:23 'For the wages of sin is death, but the gift of God is eternal life in Christ Jesus our Lord.' The next..."

"Wait a minute!" Ramon exclaimed, waving his hand.

Eric looked up and asked, "Yes?"

"Okay, I know I've sinned, that's doing wrong, isn't it?" Eric nodded. "So what's this 'eternal life' you talk about?"

"I don't know what you think happens after death, I don't know you that well, but after the body dies, there's a part of us, our soul that lives forever. That part either lives in eternal punishment or eternal happiness. The first's called 'Hell', the other's called 'Heaven'. Our sin sends us automatically to Hell, but we can live in Heaven if we accept God's gift of eternal life through His Son. Let me read you the next verse on the Roman's Road. It's 5: 8: 'But God demonstrates his own love for us in this: While we were still sinners, Christ died for us.'"

Scowling and concentrating on the words, Ramon said, "You mean He'll do that just as we are? We don't have to clean up our act?"

"Yeah, that's it! Listen to Romans 10: 9,10: '...if you confess with your mouth, "Jesus is Lord," and believe in your heart that God raised him from the dead, you will be saved. For it is with your heart that you believe and are justified, and it is with your mouth that you confess and are saved.' and the last one is 12:1,2: 'Therefore, I urge you, brothers, in view of God's mercy, to offer your bodies as living sacrifices, holy and pleasing to God - which is your spiritual worship. Do not conform any longer to the pattern of this world, but be transformed by the renewing of your mind. Then you will be able to test and approve what God's will is - his good, pleasing and perfect will.'"

"So, what you're saying is, I'm a sinner, I've done stuff that God says is wrong." Eric nodded. "But you're also saying that even while I'm sinning, God loved me enough to make His Son die to take my sin away." He pointed to the Bible and added, "But that was a long time ago! He died, what, two thousand years ago?"

"Yes, but He knew about you, Ramon. God knows everything! But you're right! That's it! Then, because He's done that, we must believe He did it for us and tell others that we believe it." Ramon saw him still turning pages until he found another place and said, "There's another verse in another place that says, 'For God so loved the world that he gave his one and only Son, that whoever believes in him shall not perish but have eternal life. For God did not send his Son into the world to condemn the world but to save the world through him.' (John 3: 16,17) You know who that 'whoever' is? It's you, it's me, it's anybody who will believe in God's free gift."

"Wow!" Ramon murmured, "That's awesome!" He couldn't lie on his back any longer he sat up, pulled his knees up and hugged them.

"Yes, it is, man. You want to tell God you believe?"

"Yeah, but what do I say?"

"Say what I say, it's kind of what my friend told me to say to God: 'Dear God, I know I'm a sinner. I've done wrong, but I've learned tonight that Your Son, Jesus, died to take away my sins and make me so I can have eternal life with You in Heaven. Thank You for taking away my sin, I believe You've done that. Amen.'"

Ramon flipped over onto his knees and put his face to his knees then he said the words Eric had said, coaching him. Moments later, he raised his head and looked at his friend. "He did it!" He grinned in the dim firelight, threw his arms out and his head back. As his eyes gazed heavenward, a shooting star streaked across the heavens. "He did it! I have peace in my heart that I've never had."

"Praise God!" Eric answered, quietly.

"Yes, praise God! Nearly all summer I've been hearing people read from the Bible and I've tried to find ways to get away, but it seemed there was never a good excuse and each time I heard someone read from the Bible it pricked me. My receptionist started almost immediately telling me I needed to be a Believer. I didn't listen at first, but her life spoke so loudly I had to listen. She's always been in that chair, but she's not bitter to God and she loves life."

"I know, I could tell from those few minutes we saw her yesterday. I could tell she's an awesome person. Being a Christian shines through her."

"Yeah, it does!" Ramon said then lay down on his bag. Again he looked at the expanse of sky and remembered the scripture another leader read. Yes, God was awesome!

Sandy found another deserted place to park her van for the night on Sunday. The shadows were long, but there seemed to be a window through the trees to the peak of a mountain beyond. The very top of the mountain seemed to be on fire because of the setting sun still glowing behind it. Sandy sat on the lift, still level with the inside of the van facing that window. Quickly, she grabbed her camera and snapped a picture, then picked up a small canvass, her charcoals and began. She knew there wouldn't be time to catch the awesome scene if she set up her easel and took the time to mix paints, she could do that later from the photo. She was sure she'd find time later on this year.

When she finished, she wheeled herself inside and closed the lift and the door. There wasn't enough light in the sky to see, but her picture was finished. Some other day, probably during the winter, she'd use her photo as a prompt and paint the picture. The charcoal was awesome she'd hang it at home. With the doors locked, she quickly fixed her supper. By now, it was dark and she wouldn't leave the light on long in the van, so she fixed her bed and lay down. She'd had a fantastic day.

Before she went to sleep, she said, "My Father in heaven, thank You for this awesome day. I've never been so happy as I've been this weekend living in Your gift of splendor. It is hard to believe when I see these awesome views that nature is groaning because of Man's sin, but You've said, so I believe. Bless Ramon and the men with him. Bring him to Yourself in Your own time. I've seen a subtle change in him in the month since I've come, but he has never said he's accepted You as his Savior. Bless Mom and Dad, Ed and Marcy. You know how much I love them. I miss them, but You know far better than I do why I'm here and they're there. Thank You for loving me enough to send Your Son as my Savior. In His Name, Amen."

She fell asleep and slept soundly. She slept well and only realized after she opened the door and was on the ground that something had visited during the night. She never left anything outside, but when she reached the ground, there were three cleanly stripped fish carcasses lying by her front passenger tire. She smiled knowing only one creature would leave such a calling card. A raccoon had visited during the night.

Because of the fish, she was sure there was a stream close by, even though she didn't hear any running water, so she followed the trail away from her van. Soon, there was a sparkling stream and off to one side was a gurgling waterfall just waiting to be painted. She hurried back for her easel and paints, knowing this would be her last painting for the weekend. She must go home after this. She sighed, she didn't want to leave these awesome scenes, but tomorrow was another day of work and she wouldn't miss it.

Roger held a dripping paint brush as he sat back on his heels. It was Thursday evening and the sun was casting long shadows across the hills behind the town. The men had finished putting all the lumber down for the ramp on Wednesday and since Roger didn't have a nine to five job through the week, he'd volunteered to paint the structure. Corky had warned him to get it stained at least twenty-four hours before it was to be used and to string something across each end so it wouldn't get walked on until Friday when it was perfectly dry. He sighed, all that was left to do was run the tape Corky had given him across the bottom end and he was finished.

Looking at the sun, he knew he hadn't finished any too soon. His neck was cramping and his knees felt like he'd been kneeling at the altar for days. He rolled off his heels onto his rear and stretched out his legs. He sighed, he wasn't sure he'd be able to stand yet. Looking back up the walk, he saw one end that glared white at him. He groaned and dipped his brush again into the stain, then crawled on his knees back up to swish some stain on the errant two by four end. He looked up and down more closely, hoping he wouldn't find any more white places. He didn't find any and he heaved a sigh of relief.

Finally, he felt like he could stand on his feet, so he drew his knees up, then pushed his hands against the ground and staggered to his feet. He knew he wasn't too old, but his knees snapped and felt like water as he tried to make them hold him up. He almost put his hand on the railing, but remembered just in time that it could still be wet. He put the lid back on the can of stain and hammered it down, then threw the paint brush into his bag where he was throwing his trash. Corky had warned him that brushes used for staining were hard to get clean he should buy a cheep one and throw it away when he finished. Finally, he reached for the roll of plastic tape that had the words: 'CAUTION KEEP OUT' printed across it and made an 'X' out of the tape across the opening. He was finally done and tomorrow was the concert. Everything he'd bought at the lumberyard was in the ramp, but he still had no idea how it would be paid for. He sighed, that would be a worry for another day.

As Roger put the last staple into the caution tape, Brad from the hardware store came out and called, "So, you're done finally?"

Roger made a face. "I reckon so. I thought I'd never get to that last board, but I guess I did. Not any too soon, the sun's going down."

Brad lived around the corner on a back street, but he'd brought in a load today, so as he walked to his truck, he said, "You got that right! So the concert's tomorrow? What time?"

Roger rolled up the caution tape, picked up the stapler, the stain and his trash and put it all into the back of his Jeep. "It's at seven thirty. It should be good, I've heard her play."

Brad grunted. "Too bad I don't close till eight on Fridays."

From beside the driver's door, Roger said, "I'm sure she won't be done by eight. She's got music for an hour and a half with an intermission thrown in."

Brad nodded. "I'll talk my wife into comin' and savin' me a seat. Achally, she's into that kind of stuff."

Roger swung into his seat and as he stuck the key into the ignition, he said, "You'd better do that, I'm sure the place'll be full. We never had such a thing here since I've lived here. See you, I got livestock to feed." Brad saluted him and opened his truck door, but Roger was intent on getting home to his house.

Roger turned the key and his several-years-old Jeep groaned to life. One day soon, after the lumber was paid for, he'd probably have to buy new wheels. Only seconds later, his stomach reminded him he'd painted right through lunch time and all he'd put into his mouth had been caffeine laced soft drinks. He knew better, but it was easy and handy to dash across the street and snag a can from Brad's ready supply.

He parked beside his house and his faithful mutt came to the side of his Jeep, his whole rear end wagging. Absently, Roger reached down and scratched his ears. He went inside and the red light on his answering machine was flashing. He hit the retrieve button and a pleasing voice said, "Hi, this is Sandy Bernard. I never thought to ask before and I guess it's a little late to ask now, but was the piano in your church tuned lately? I'm sorry I didn't think to ask sooner. See you tomorrow. Bye."

With each word, Roger's eyes grew larger and his chin dropped. The piano in the church tuned? Who would know? He sure didn't. He didn't play piano and they never used it during their worship hours. For all he knew, it sat in the corner collecting dust. He'd never thought about it. He didn't have much of an ear, but maybe he'd better go run his fingers up and down some keys. He put some food down for the cat who was winding himself around his legs, then hopped back in his Jeep and hurried back to town.

It was dark now, but Roger ran up the five steps and opened the front door of the church. It was even darker in the building and since they didn't have evening services, he had to hunt for the switch for the lights that lit the sides of the auditorium. Groping along the wall, he finally found the switch and flipped it on. He let the door close behind him; he wasn't too keen on someone hearing him plink on the piano keys. He went to the front and lifted the lid over the keys and noticed immediately that the ivories and ebonies hadn't been cleaned in a very long time they were coated with greasy dust. He guessed that answered Sandy question. If nobody had played it, so that the ivories were that dirty, it hadn't been tuned in forever.

He pulled out his bandana that he'd used all day to wipe his sweaty forehead and swiped it along the keys. When he had the dust gone, he stretched his fingers to be eight keys apart. He knew enough about a piano that notes eight keys apart were the same sound only higher or lower. Carefully, with thumbs and little fingers of both hands, he pressed down four keys, they all sounded like the same sound only higher and lower, then moved up one key. To his untrained ear, it sounded okay, but Sandy would probably cringe.

He moved up five notes, but the sixth note there were only three sounds. He took his hands off and tried working his finger over the 'A' note, the one above middle 'C'. Even though he pressed it several times, there was no sound. He thought of the piece he'd heard a part of that afternoon and knew she'd have to use that note. Not knowing what else to do, he raised the cover of the old upright and peered over the edge. Much to his surprise, a mouse was hugging the string and when he hit the key, a hammer bounced off the mouse's back.

Roger chuckled. "Love that note, do you, buddy?" For some strange reason, the little creature didn't answer him.

He left the top up then pulled the piano bench up close. He climbed up and stuck his hand inside. The mouse didn't move, but it hung onto the strings fiercely. Roger had to pry the paws away, but when he pulled the dead creature out, it hadn't been dead long, the body was not decomposed. After he disposed of the mouse, he went back and continued his four finger exploration up and down the keys. He decided that since the concert was tomorrow night, the sounds the piano made were what people would hear who came, whether they were true or not.

When he left the church, he crossed the street and in the street light in front of Brad's store, copied down the number from Sandy's picture in his window. He drove home, his stomach growling all the way, and parked beside his dark house. The thought dashed through his mind, would he ever come home to a house that had lights on because there was a wife and kids already there? He sighed. As far as he knew, Sandy Bernard was the only young single woman in town right now and he'd been 'Johnny come lately' as far as she was concerned.

After he opened a can of soup and poured the contents into a sauce pan on the stove, he dialed the number he'd written down. A cheerful voice said, "Hello?"

"Hi, Sandy, it's Roger. I never thought to check the piano until I got your message. I'm sorry about that. Anyway, I'm back from checking it out." He grinned, should he tell her about the mouse? Sure, why not!

"Is it okay?"

"I don't really know how you tell, but I do know about octaves, so I ran up and down the notes. I, umm, came to the key five above middle 'C' and it didn't play."

"Oh, no! You mean the 'A'?"

"Yeah, I think that's it. Anyway, I hit it several times and nothing happened, so I lifted the lid to check out why it was quiet and a mouse had wrapped himself around the strings."

He heard a gasp and a thin little voice said, "A…a mouse?"

Grinning even more broadly, he said, "Yeah, well, I tried to coax him out, but you know how mice are, he'd have none of it, so I had to reach down in there…"

Another gasp and the little voice asked, "Did… did he bite you?"

By now, Roger had all he could do to keep his voice serious. "Well, no, he was sort of docile, he'd been dead a day or two, I think."

Sandy's voice was back to normal, when she said, "For goodness sake, Roger, you had me going there for a minute!" She laughed and Roger laughed with her. Finally, when her giggles stopped, she said, "So now all the notes make sound? Do they sound well together? You know I'll be putting a lot together."

"To answer your question from my machine, Sandy, I don't think the piano's been tuned recently, but I think it'll all go together pretty well. Besides, who beside you is an expert?"

Sandy sighed, "Roger, probably no one. It's just when you play a concert you want everything to be perfect. I wish I'd have thought about it before, I'd have called the man who tuned my piano when I first came to tune that one, but I never thought."

"I'm sure it'll be fine, Sandy, nobody around here's going to jump up and run out if they hear a sour note, I'm sure." Changing the subject and turning off the fire under his soup, Roger asked, "So, has Ramon showed his face yet?"

"He had a three day back to back with Labor Day. He brought one group back late on Monday and took a group out at eight on Tuesday. They were supposed to get back about supper time today. From his schedule, he has tomorrow off and then heads out again on Saturday for another week long hike."

Roger shook his head and took a second to blow on his soup. "The man's burning the candle at both ends! He'll be so burned out by the end of the season he'll burn his backpack before he comes inside after that last trip!"

"I know, I've told him that, too. A man who wants to be a guide too went on the Labor Day hike. Maybe he won't be so covered up next year."

Sandy had such a pleasing voice that Roger wanted to keep her talking, but he knew he'd want a lot more if he did, so he blew on his soup again and said, "I'll see you tomorrow. By the way, how early do you want to be inside?"

"Let's say six thirty, would that be okay with you?"

"Sure! I'll have the place open. See you then."

Sandy hung up and turned to her perfectly tuned piano. One last time she placed her black pressure pouch on her chair and started her metronome. Without any music in front of her, she began to play her Chopin piece. She had it all memorized, but there was one section that had so many notes and intricate fingerings that she had a hard time keeping up with the metronome. She came to the part and this time sailed right through it. When she came to the end, there was sweat sitting on her upper lip, but she'd finished the piece perfectly.

"It's about time!" she grumbled. Up to this point Mr. Chopin had probably been turning over in his grave, but this time, he surely lay back down and sighed with satisfaction. She could only hope he'd be pleased tomorrow night, too. She shook her head, how long had it taken her to get it right? She needed to get cracking on new stuff more often!

Ramon smiled half-heartedly at his hikers as they crowded around their cars in the parking lot. It had been a rough six days, since the Saturday before Labor Day. He'd had a great time with his friends and Duncan, but the hike had been strenuous, one he was glad he didn't take every time he led a group. He'd been tired, but all the time he'd had before the next hike was spent washing, drying and repacking his clothes, eating two meals and sleeping eight hours in his bed. He hadn't made one phone call, even though he'd wanted to hear Sandy's voice.

As the sun crept toward the hills behind his house, the parking lot emptied and all that was left was his own truck parked to the side of the house. He picked up his backpack by the straps, found his hidden key and went into the solitude of his office. There were messages Sandy had left him sitting on the blotter on his desk. He dropped the pack at the corner of his desk and slouched into his chair, eager to read Sandy's notes. Of course, one of them said to call his mom. He sighed maybe he'd do that on the second Tuesday next week.

After reading all the notes, he took his pack into the other part of the house straight to the laundry room. It hadn't rained, but it had been hot. Even after emptying the clothes into the washer the pack smelled of sweat. Before he started the machine, he emptied all the pockets and threw the pack into the washer. Thank goodness the thing was washable. With Sandy still on his mind, he fixed some supper and sat down to eat. Tomorrow was her concert and he was MC.

He hadn't seen Sandy since Saturday morning when he'd led his men back from their parked vehicle to where Sandy was painting. He'd missed her and he had some news he had to share with her. He looked at the clock and shrugged, so it was dark and a bit late to go visiting, especially a single man to a single woman, but that was too bad, he wanted to see her too badly.

He waited for the washer to stop, took the load from it to the dryer and started the machine. He pulled the truck keys from the peg and left by the office door. Sandy had a porch light, after he knocked he'd step back so she could see him. He had to see her and tell her his news. He was excited to tell her and he was sure she'd be excited to hear it.

He pulled onto Isabel's parking lot and pulled in front of Sandy's van. All the weariness he'd felt from the hike was gone. He bounded up the ramp of Sandy's cabin and heard her playing the most beautiful music he could remember hearing. He stood close to the window and watched her fingers fly over the keys and saw the rhythmic movement of her shoulder as she used the sustaining pedal. This lady was an awesome person, he knew she was a beautiful person, not only her face, but her... the lady herself was beautiful. And now he had also experienced what she had.

Sandy raised her hands from the keys and immediately there was a knock on the door. It was dark out, who could it be? She turned off the metronome and went to the door, but before she opened it, she turned on the porch light and looked out the window. Ramon stood back from the door smiling at her. She grinned and threw the door open.

"Ramon! It's good to see you! Come in. Aren't you exhausted after so many trips?"

He walked in, still with the huge grin on his face but went straight to her couch, sank down onto it and sighed, "Yeah, I'm pretty tired, but something happened that I have to tell you about." Even as he spoke, the whir of her chair motor started. In only seconds she was beside him, looking at him intently. "It was over Labor Day, but there wasn't time before I had to leave again, but I couldn't wait any longer to tell you."

She wheeled so close her footrest almost touched his ankle. The anticipation level was high in her voice, as she asked, "What is it?" Her elbows were resting on the armrests of her chair, her hands dangling above her lap.

Ramon leaned toward her, reached out and took her hands then he looked into her eyes and said, "Sandy, you know I've had no time for God, all my life." He sighed, "I've scoffed and said I'd never have anything to do with Him." She nodded, her hands squeezing his. "But I've heard what you've said since you came. I've taken several church groups this summer and that one where the woman was injured really got to me. They had devotions each night and two times the pastor read a Psalm that was so relevant and powerful I couldn't ignore it."

He looked down at their joined hands, then back up to her eyes. As usual, they were sparkling, there was a grin on her face as if she knew what he was about to say. She always made it so easy to talk to her, to tell her anything. She felt him squeeze her hands she squeezed back, encouraging him to tell her.

He took a deep breath and said, "One of the guys who hiked with the group over Labor Day just became a Christian a week before. He took me down the Romans Road and I believed and now I have peace in my heart."

Sandy totally surprised him by yanking her hands out of Ramon's and holding out her arms to him. Ramon's secret desire ever since August had been to hold this lovely lady in his arms. When he realized her silent plea, he wasted no time in coming to his feet and circling her shoulders while she hugged him tightly. She smelled like sunshine, gardenias, outdoors, anything that was beautiful and perfect, she was the epitome!

"Ramon! Oh, I'm thrilled! Yes, God is truly working! I've prayed for Him to bring you to Himself and He's used many people to do that. Praise God!"

Against her hair, he murmured, "Yes, praise God."

After holding her for several seconds, he realized how uncomfortable it was, besides, he really wanted to kiss her and it wouldn't happen if they stayed like this. After several minutes holding her he backed out of her arms, but kept his hands on her shoulders and looked deeply into her eyes. She had her arms out, but she looked up at him totally perplexed, her wide smile had slipped a little. His eyes found hers, he didn't know what his told her, but he had to try he wanted to hold her so badly. Not knowing how else to ask, he blurted out, "Sandy, I guess I'll have to blurt this out, because I don't know how else to do it, but does it hurt you, or would you have discomfort to sit on the couch beside me?"

Her smile came back full force, as she exclaimed, "No! Oh, no! Of course not, Ramon, I'm a little squatty, that's all."

She lifted the removable armrest, preparing to shift out of her chair, but Ramon's strong arms moved quickly to her, one to her shoulders the other under her legs. The armrest clattered to the floor, but neither of them noticed. He lifted her effortlessly and set her on the couch then he sat down beside her. He didn't take his arm away from her shoulders instead, he drew her back against his side.

His breath stirred the hair beside her ear and sent shivers down her back, as he said, "Do you mind, Sandy?"

She turned and looked at him, before she said, "Why, no! This is fine." Her voice became a whisper, as she said, "In fact, this is super!"

Pulling her tightly against him, he also whispered, "I think so, too."

Sandy didn't know what to do with her hands she didn't want them to be idle in her lap. She felt his arm around her shoulders, his hand on her upper arm. Finally, she saw his other hand resting on his leg, so she picked it up and held it between both of hers. It was much larger than hers and bronze, instead of the lily white of hers. However, the minute she did, it felt like she'd picked up a live wire instead of his hand. She looked from their hands to his face in confusion, but his eyes had that same darkness she'd seen before and didn't know what it was.

"Did you feel that?" she gasped.

"Yes, I felt it."

"I only took your hand, what does it mean?"

"I'll tell you what it means to me, Sandy."

Confusion bright in her eyes, she asked, "What does it mean to you? Ramon, I have no idea what it means."

Ramon brought his lips right beside her hair so that the words moved the curls, as he said, "To me it means that I'm very, very attracted to you, Sandy."

Her eyes grew huge, as the words sank in. She turned her head and stared at him, but finally, she murmured, "Really? You are? But...but how can you be?"

The hand she held grasped hers tightly and his other hand held her face so she couldn't move it. He saw that confusion he'd seen in her eyes before. "Sandy! You're a beautiful woman. I noticed that the first time I saw you. As I got to know you, I began to see the inner beauty that you have and that radiates from you, through everything you say and do. There is absolutely nothing about you that is not beautiful, nothing! You live each day to the fullest, you are not bitter. I could go on and on!"

Shaking her head slowly, but still keeping her eyes on his, she whispered, "But Ramon, I'm paralyzed from the waist down. I have no feeling below my waist. I sit in a wheelchair, it's not pretty, in fact, it's ugly."

He pulled his hand from hers and put it gently on her cheek. Looking deeply into her eyes, he shook his head. "Sandy, your wheelchair makes no difference to me. I forgot about it that day you were painting my picture there at the pull-off. It makes no difference to me at all. I don't see a 'cripple' or even a handicapped woman, I see the most lovely, vivacious, creative, fun-loving woman I've ever met in my life. Sandy, you're not handicapped, you're more alive than many women who have total use of their legs. I don't want to ever hear you talk about that chair again!" he ended fiercely.

She couldn't drag her eyes away, as she said, "I won't, not ever."

His eyes dropped from hers down to her lips, then back to her eyes. "Sandy," he whispered, "could I... would it be all right if I kissed you?"

"You... you want to kiss me?" she gasped.

"Yes, I want to very much." He chuckled. "I've wanted to kiss you very much for quite a while, but I knew I had no right."

Unconsciously, she licked her lips. "Daddy's the only man who's ever kissed me. I... I'm not sure I know how to kiss someone. Daddy only ever kissed me on the cheek." She looked down at his lips and saw that they were full, dark red. She looked back up and her eyes twinkled. "I have a feeling yours'll be a bit different, though."

He grinned and the merriment came through in his words. "I should hope so! Want to try it to find out and see if you like it?"

"Yes," she whispered, breathlessly.

Without another word, his hand left her cheek and moved to the back of her head, tangling in her hair. His other arm brought her all the way around possessively. She hardly noticed, because his lips slowly moved toward hers. As he came closer, she couldn't keep looking at him, her eyelids closed as she anticipated his kiss.

THIRTEEN

As she said, it was different from any kiss she'd had. No one had kissed her lips. Her family kissed, but only on their cheeks, they were light and lasted momentarily. Ramon's kiss at first was firm, but the new sensations went throughout her body, sending responses from every place where she could feel. Without knowing when, her hands left her lap and moved slowly up his chest, then circled his neck and her fingers moved into his hair. He groaned when he felt them, she had such a hold over him, but there was nothing more precious than that hold!

She nearly lost her breath, but finally he drew his lips away. Her eyes flew open as she dragged in a long breath. "Oh, my!" she said.

Brushing her lips again with his, he murmured against them, "My feelings exactly, Sandy. Oh, my!" He leaned his forehead against hers while they caught their breath. He held her, loving the feel of this lovely lady in his arms.

After several minutes had passed, he kissed her again, but not until they were breathless, then pulled his hand from her hair and leaned back against the cushions, bringing her with him. He didn't want to stop kissing her, but decided to say, "Was that one of the pieces you're playing for your concert tomorrow?"

"Yes, it's the one I'm playing after the intermission. I decided instead of playing all pieces I knew really well, I'd conquer a new one. That was the first time I'd played it up to speed and without a mistake. I was getting a little annoyed with Mr. Chopin for making the piece so hard," her last sentence showed her annoyance

Ramon laughed. "Tell me, how long's that man been dead?"

"I don't know, a few hundred years." She grinned. "Are you all ready to be MC?"

He let a shudder move up his back and said, "Don't remind me! My mom said she'd come just to see me stutter."

"Stutter!"

Leaning his head back on the couch, he said, "Yeah, she came to a program our seventh grade class put on and I had the hardest time getting the words out of my three line speech. She doesn't think I'll do any better this time."

Confidently, she said, "Oh, for goodness sake! I don't believe that for a minute! Roger came by a few days ago and picked up my list of pieces to make a program. There's one on the table in the kitchen, if you want to see it."

He looked over and saw the folded paper, but he said, "It'd be nice to see it, but I'm holding this lovely lady and I'd rather do that."

Sandy laid her head back on his chest. It felt so right, she could hear his strong, athletic heart beating, but it felt like hers was beating in the same rhythm. She captured his free hand again and said, "I'd rather have you do that, too."

They sat silently for a few minutes, but then Ramon said, "I suppose I'd better think about going home. Sitting on this soft couch is letting *rigor mortis* set in. I should get to my bed before it totally takes over this body." He pulled his hand from hers again, curled his finger under her chin and raised her face. "That kiss was super do you think I could have another? You know, it would be like a promise for next time?"

Gladly, with a wonderful smile just for him, her eyes sparkling, she raised her face and said, "Ramon, yes! Yes!"

Without hesitation his lips found hers. It was firm again, but again it sent hot sensations through her body. She wondered briefly if they were going through the parts of her body she'd never felt in her life. Would her toes tingle? Surely they would, they had to, the way the rest of her was tingling. Before she knew what was happening, Ramon's tongue slid along her lower lip. She gasped and her lips parted, that sent a whole new raft of sensations through her. It was so powerful she shook all over. Talk about tingling!

When finally Ramon lifted his head, their breath was coming in heavy breaths. When Sandy could finally open her eyes, she was looking into his and finally, she understood why his eyes became so much darker. She remembered that look from when they'd been in the closet. He'd told her he'd wanted to kiss her for a very long time. Could it be even since then? Was Isabel right? Did Ramon really love her? Maybe it was the late hour and he was tired from being on the trail so much. Surely he didn't love her, did he?

Ramon still held her, but looked at her clock hanging over the archway. It was big and bold, with a white face and every number black, not hard to see. He didn't have to look long to know that it was late and he'd been on a trail all day and most of the time for over a week. He sighed and said, "I guess I've stayed as long as I should, probably longer. Could I take your program to learn the names of the pieces and the men's names who wrote them? It wouldn't be too good if I called him 'Mr. Chop in'."

Sandy laughed. "Sure you can take it. I know how things are going, but I'm real sure you won't be calling him 'Mr. Chop in' he'd probably turn over in his grave if you did." She put her face up again and kissed him on the lips again. "Thanks for tonight, Ramon. It's been the best I've ever had."

As he stood up, he squeezed her shoulder and said, "That's the same for me, too." He looked from her to her chair and said, "Should I put you back in your chair?"

"It'd be great if you don't mind, I need to get to the bathroom and into the bedroom."

"I'll do that." He picked her up almost like a feather and set her in her chair, then picked up the armrest from the floor.

He smiled at her and brushed her lips again, then headed for the door. "Sleep well, Sandy, I'll see you tomorrow."

"Yes, you will!"

Roger carried the milk pail onto the back porch and heard the phone ring. It nearly made him slosh some of the milk from the pail, even though it wasn't half full. He wasn't used to hearing the phone this early in the morning. Who called anyone before businesses opened at eight? Quickly, he pushed open the back door into the kitchen and hurried across the room to grab the receiver before the answering machine picked it up.

Breathlessly, he answered, "Hello?"

Instantly a clipped, rather British, no-nonsense voice said, "Roger Clemens, is he there?"

"This is Roger. What can I do for you?"

"Listen, I'm sitting here looking at this church building that's supposed to be open for me to tune a piano. I waited for several minutes then checked in the gas station and the man said to call Roger Clemens and gave me this number. I'm a very busy man, when can you arrive? I don't like to be kept waiting when I have an appointment."

Smelling the manure on his barn shoes and knowing he'd only thrown on the dirty clothes from yesterday to milk his one cow, he said, "Yes, sir. Give me twenty minutes, I can't make it there any quicker than that."

"I'll be waiting!" he exclaimed.

The dial tone hummed in his ear even before Roger could pull the receiver away. "Well! You have a good day, too! Yeah, and thanks for disrupting my plans for the day. It's real kind of you. I'll see you in twenty minutes." he grumbled as he hung the receiver back on the wall and shook his head.

With a sigh, knowing that to keep the milk from spoiling he had to take care of it immediately, he set the pail on the counter, found his strainer and a gallon jug and poured the milk through the strainer into the jug, yanked open the refrigerator door and shoved the jug in, then slammed the door as he headed for the back door to pull off his barn boots. From there he started stripping clothes from his body as he headed for the shower. With another sigh, he wondered where the simple 'good ol' days' had gone.

Under the shower he scrubbed his hair and a thought hit him. Was Sandy that well known, was she some celebrity that had come to Vansville incognito that she could command a piano tuner to drop everything and come tune his piano? As far as he knew, no one had even thought about an out-of-tune piano until yesterday, yesterday evening to be exact! Besides, who was supposed to have called him to have the church open so this man could tune it? Since he lived alone, nobody answered his questions. He tore out of his house still buttoning his shirt. He was glad he usually left the keys in the Jeep.

Twenty-two minutes after hanging up, he wheeled into town and saw a new truck parked in front of the church. The man sitting in the driver's seat had his left arm up, obviously inspecting his watch. Roger sighed and pulled behind the truck. Both men exited their vehicles at the same time, but the man in front reached back for a briefcase from the passenger seat.

"So, you're Roger Clemens," he said, as Roger walked up.

"Yes, I am. I wasn't aware that I was to have the church open this morning. Who was supposed to have called me?"

The man looked at Roger as if he had no intelligence at all. "A friend of mine, Derek Casbah. He said there's a concert here tonight and he's sure the piano sounds dreadful. He cannot abide an out-of-tune piano." Using his hand to usher Roger ahead of him, he said, "Well, be about it! Get the door open."

Roger stared at the man and his jaw dropped, then snapped it shut, his teeth making a resounding crack, finally he nodded. Ramon's step-dad had ordered the piano tuned? Roger swallowed and said, "I'll get that door right away. How long does it take?"

Following close behind Roger, the man said, "It depends how bad it sounds. I'll have to listen to it before I can tell you."

Roger opened the door and said, "Perhaps you could tell me your name?"

Arrogantly, he said, "I'm Christopher Jehling. I work out of Blairsville. Of course, I have my own business."

Roger didn't offer his hand, he was sure the man wouldn't take it anyway. "I'm pleased to meet you, Mr. Jehling. As you can see, the piano is up there in the front."

Peering through the dim sanctuary, Mr. Jehling gasped and said, "Someone is going to play a piano concert on that old thing?"

Trying not to sound affronted, Roger flipped on the lights and started walking toward the piano and said, "It seems so. That is the only one in the building and this building is the biggest place to hold a concert in Vansville."

"Well!" Mr. Jehling sighed and started walking toward the instrument. "This makes my job *infinitely* harder and I'm sure much more time consuming."

Roger didn't comment. One thing in the piano's favor, that Mr. Jehling didn't know, a mouse had been removed last night. The man thumped his briefcase down on the piano bench and opened it, at least the man couldn't complain about the dust on the keys that Roger had cleaned away yesterday. Immediately he opened the cover and did what Roger had done yesterday, starting with his right thumb on middle 'C' and his left thumb an octave lower, then with his little fingers making four octaves sound together. They sounded pretty good to Roger.

Mr. Jehling moved up a note, then another and Roger saw a shudder work down the man's spine. "Oh, my! Do you know when this was last tuned?"

Roger shook his head. "I have no idea. I've only worked with this church for five years, but I've not known anything to be done to it in that time."

"Oh, my!"

He turned to his briefcase and pulled out a cell phone, punched in one key, then held the instrument to his ear. Seconds later, he said, "Elizabeth, you'll need to call all my morning appointments and cancel. Set them up for some other day." There was a pause. "This instrument Derek wanted a rush job on will take at least four hours to do." He pulled the tiny phone from his ear and snapped it shut. Turning to Roger, he said, "You heard what I said to my secretary, I'm sure it'll take at least four hours. Surely, you can leave and come back?"

"Sure! I'll be glad to, Mr. Jehling."

Roger hurried toward the main door, went out and closed the door. Already, Mr. Jehling was banging on the keys and Roger was glad to be outside of the door from his noise. He waved to Brad who peered out the door to see what was going on across the street, but didn't cross the street to tell him. He jumped back into his Jeep and headed back home. His stomach was protesting the fact that it hadn't had any breakfast as yet. Usually he had some of that warm milk on his cereal, but that wouldn't happen today. Maybe he'd have a fresh egg omelet instead.

He chuckled. So they'd get the piano tuned at the expense of the richest man in town, would that he'd also pay for the ramp they'd completed the day before. He sighed, knowing that unless he asked for a special offering in church, it was his baby. He might as well bite the bullet and take those odd jobs people asked him about, that would help pay for that new pile of lumber in front of the church. He could only hope all those people he'd told he didn't know how to be a handyman would forget he'd said that. After all, he now owned a hammer.

A warm, fuzzy dream woke Sandy Friday morning. Since it was Friday, Sandy went to Ramon's office as usual. After kissing her several times last evening, she wondered what he would do this morning. She hoped he wouldn't try to ignore what they'd done, she'd found his kisses to be the most wonderful happening in her life so far. She turned the corner onto the parking lot and parked in her place. His truck was parked in its usual place beside the house. There weren't any other vehicles on the lot. As she started to activate the controls from the inside, the office door opened. A smiling Ramon greeted her as she lowered the lift from its travel position. She found her own smile was crinkling her skin.

As soon as she was on the lift, he reached up and pushed the button to bring it down to the pavement. "Hi!" he said, "You look great!"

She rolled off the lift and turned toward the back of the van with her key extended and said, "Hi! You look great, too. You must feel more rested when you've slept in your own bed."

"Something like that." He wasn't about to tell her about all the dreams that woke him up nearly every hour all night. It made him wonder if she'd had any, not that he'd ask or anything.

He walked beside her until they reached the door, then he stepped ahead and opened it for her. He followed her inside and closed the door tightly behind him. He didn't even let her move to the desk before he snagged her around the shoulders and bent over, the humming of her chair motor stopped instantly. Bringing his head to her level and still smiling, he looked into her eyes. When he saw acceptance, his heart ratcheted up at least three notches before he claimed her soft, warm lips and heard a contented sigh. Was that his or hers?

After several minutes of savoring their kiss, he pulled his lips from hers and whispered, "I've thought about doing that ever since I woke up." She didn't have time to comment before the phone rang. However, Ramon couldn't help but notice how red and kissable those lips were. He grinned, his probably were, too.

Since he was standing up, Ramon sighed and reached for the receiver, leaving his hand on her shoulder and barked, "Hello?"

"Hi," Duncan said, "I figured it'd be Sandy who answered."

Wanting to brush his shoulder, because he felt that little green varmint sitting there grinning at him, Ramon answered, "She's here, but I was closer. What's up, Duncan?"

"When's your next trip?"

"I leave in the morning at eight for a five day."

"Could I tag along?"

"Sure! No problem, I'll be glad for you to go." Remembering Duncan's reaction to Eric on their Labor Day trip, he chuckled and said, "Duncan, you may want to know it's a church youth group who's going this time."

There was a short pause before he answered, "No problem, if they leave me alone, I'll leave them alone. We'll get along fine that way."

"I'm sure they will, but some of these church groups have devotions after supper. So I'll see you tomorrow morning?"

"I'm planning to come to Sandy's concert tonight. I'll see you then."

"Hey, that's super!"

By now, Sandy was pulling out Ramon's appointment book and was turned from him. His hand actually did reach to his shoulder and give it a swipe. When he realized what he'd done, he grunted, "Sure! In a place that small I'm sure we'll see each other." Grinning just a little, he added, "Remember it's at the church."

Ignoring that, Duncan said, "Didn't you say the concert's at seven thirty?"

"It sure is and I'm the MC."

"Great! I'll be there."

When Ramon hung up, Sandy looked up and asked, "Do you have a sore shoulder? You've been rubbing it ever since I pulled around your desk."

Ramon realized his hand was still on his shoulder so he gave it one last good swipe, then dropped it quickly and said, "No, I guess I had an itch."

Not looking at him, but at the appointment book, she said, "So that was Duncan? He wants to go on your next hike? I guess that's good, he'll get acquainted with the area this year."

"Yes." Not wanting to talk about Duncan at all, he changed the subject and asked, "What do you know about computers?"

She shrugged, then looked up with her usual smile and said, "They're something I'd like to learn about. They're the thing of the present and I'm sure of the future, but I've had no experience with them. There is not one in the house I lived in for almost twenty-five years."

Coming up behind her and laying his hands on her shoulders, he said, "Hmm. I guess you're as illiterate as I am. No one at your home has one?"

"My dad's a mail carrier with a walking route and has a woodworking hobby, my mom's never worked outside the home, she writes letters long hand. My brother's in his first year of grad school and does his computer work at the university when he needs to and my sister is in nursing school. She stays in the nurse's residence except for an occasional day off, but she doesn't bring school work home with her. No, we've never had a computer in the house."

Ramon sighed, "Duncan just about has me convinced I need to get a computer. He's become familiar with this area by punching in some cities and towns, as well as highways and country roads and using those things as coordinates to show what he wants to know about the area on his computer. He's showed me some things that can be done with it that includes setting up the schedule for next season. Believe it or not, those maps show trails, so we can probably set up new trails for next year's hikes."

"It sounds interesting, Ramon."

"It was. Umm, since you're staying here in Vansville, could I ask if you'd be interested in working with us some on this after October?"

"Sure! I have no problem with that. I think it'll be interesting. So is Duncan staying around in the area over the winter?"

"He said he doesn't have a place he calls home, so he said he would."

"Will he find a place to live close by?"

Ramon cleared his throat. "I think he's thinking about asking Isabel if he can rent one of her cabins for several months."

Sandy nodded. "I'm sure she'll be glad for the steady income over the winter, she told me her heat bills nearly eat her up. Why did you tell him it was a church youth group you're taking? Was that supposed to mean something? And then you said the concert was at the church. Was that important?"

Ramon shook his head then sat in his office chair beside the desk. "He wasn't totally rude to Eric about his beliefs on the hike, but I could tell he had no time for any religious talk. He made sure he was not hiking close to Eric once he learned he was a Christian. If I hiked with Eric, Duncan didn't speak to me until I moved away from him."

Sandy scowled, a totally foreign expression, and said, "He's someone we need to add to our prayer list." She grinned and said, "Of course, I can take you off, but if he's living in Isabel's cabin, he'll automatically be on her prayer list." She looked up at Ramon and said, "I think we need to add Roger to that list, too."

Incredulous, Ramon swallowed then exclaimed, "Roger! The preacher? On your prayer list? What for?"

Very seriously, no smile on her face, Sandy said, "Isabel said his talks on Sunday morning could be readings from the Reader's Digest. When he came by for my list of pieces to make the programs, I wasn't impressed with his philosophy as being very Christian." She cleared her throat. "I'm afraid I was pretty blunt and laid it on the line. He never assured me he agreed with me or told me he was a Believer. I don't think the people who go to his church have ever heard Scripture read or the gospel preached from his pulpit."

"Wow!"

Sandy nodded. "Yeah, my thoughts precisely."

Ramon pulled his hand reluctantly from hers and said, "How about a glass of iced tea while you sift through the messages on the answering machine?"

Sandy grinned at him. "Sounds like you need a caffeine fix. I'll have one with you."

"Great! I'll be back in a second."

While he was in the hallway on the way to the kitchen, the phone rang, so Sandy picked up the office phone and said, "DeLord's Hiking…"

"Hi, Sandy, it's Roger. You'll never guess what I just did!"

"Okay, you'd better tell me."

"I let a Mr. Jehling into the church so he could tune the piano."

"**What!?**"

"Yeah. A Mr. Jehling from Blairsville demanded I rush into town and open the church so he could tune the piano for the concert tonight. He's there now."

"But we only talked last night about whether it was in tune or not!"

"Exactly! When I asked, he said Mr. Casbah insisted he tune the piano today because there was a concert tonight and he couldn't stand an out-of-tune piano. I just about fell over."

Smiling at the young man who had just returned to the office, holding two glasses, Sandy said, "My, my, my! I'm sure that'll be news to my boss."

Ramon stepped back into the office as Sandy spoke and scowled. Was she talking about him? He didn't feel like her boss, not at all! He set her glass of tea on the blotter and plopped down onto the chair he'd left momentarily, planning on being quiet enough that he could possibly hear the rest of the conversation. Who in the world could she be talking about that she'd call him her boss?

Roger chuckled. "You do that, I'm sure he doesn't know anything about it."

"I will. You'll have the place open at six thirty?"

"I sure will. Is Ramon all rehearsed for his job?"

Sandy looked at him and grinned. "I don't know. He told me he stuttered the last time he got up in front of people."

"Ramon, stutter?" Roger laughed. "Oh, great! I'm glad I'll be there to see if he does. So I'll see you tonight."

"Yes. Thanks for that piece of information, Roger. See you then."

Sandy hung up and Ramon said, "Your boss?"

Nodding, Sandy asked, "You know a Mr. Jehling?"

"Never heard of him."

Her eyes twinkling and a smile twitching her lips, Sandy said, "Roger said he had a call early and had to rush into town to open the church for a Mr. Jehling who had been sent to tune the piano for tonight's concert by a Mr. Casbah who can't abide an out-of-tune piano. You say you don't know this Mr. Jehling?"

There was a young man in the office at DeLord's who had to swallow before he said, "I know the Mr. Casbah you speak of and I know he's into classical music and he takes Mom to many concerts as far away as Atlanta, but I didn't know he'd go so far as to send a man out just to tune Roger's piano. Wow!" he said, shaking his head. "That is truly amazing!" He looked at his watch. "Even now he's there?"

"It seems so."

Ramon shook his head and took a sip from his glass. "That is unbelievable! You haven't even met my step-dad, have you?"

Sandy nodded. "That day your mom rammed her car into the tree in front of my cabin, he came. He introduced himself and we talked a minute. He wasn't rude, just cool. Of course, he had to be concerned about Millie."

Ramon shrugged. "Mmm, maybe a little."

"Ramon, don't they get along?"

"I really don't know. I haven't been in their house in three years, maybe longer. Derek and I don't get along, so I don't make the effort to be friendly. Of course, you know Mom, she's forever coming by to see me or calling, so I don't have to make the effort to see her or go there."

"She hasn't been by since her accident."

"I threw her off the place that day, but Derek said he wasn't getting her a car right away, either. Even if he fixes her Jag she probably won't drive it."

Sandy shook her head. "She's a very unhappy woman."

"She is that and she tries to make everyone else she knows unhappy along with her. She's been unhappy for as long as I can remember."

Putting her hand over his, she said, "I tried to be a friend to her that day after her wreck, but she only sat in the car and screamed at me."

Ramon shook his head, set down his empty glass. Coming to her, he smiled, took her glass, setting it beside his. "Let's not talk about her, on such a beautiful day there have to be more pleasant things to talk about." He whispered, "Would a kiss be okay right now?"

Immediately, Sandy gave him a fantastic smile and lifted her face. "Of course!" She licked her lips and whispered, "You kisses are addicting, Ramon."

Ramon's arm slid around her shoulders, but her hands moved to his neck. Their lips came together and her eyelids closed. Just before his lips settled on hers, he whispered, "Sandy, you are so lovely. You make my heart sing!" She couldn't have replied, his lips claimed hers and caused any words to fly right out of her head.

They came up for air once, but only long enough to take a deep breath before his claimed hers again. For some miraculous reason, the phone stayed quiet. His tongue tentatively ventured from his mouth and ran along her lower lip. She gasped and he touched her teeth with his tongue. She didn't open her teeth, but her hands grasped his hair in an almost death-like grip. Neither of them noticed the movement on the parking lot. They weren't even aware of the car door slamming. The first thing that brought them back to reality was the door, slamming back against the wall. Ramon reluctantly pulled his lips from Sandy's and they both looked toward the person standing in the doorway.

It could have been the Georgia version of the female storm cloud.

"What are you doing?" Millie screamed.

Unrepentant, Ramon said, "I'm kissing Sandy. Good morning, Mom. What brings you here? Why don't you come in and close the door. We don't need to cool all outside, you know."

She took one step, grabbed the doorknob and yanked the door, making it slam behind her. With fire in her eyes and venom in her voice she said, "I knew you were home. I didn't think she'd be here, too."

Keeping his arms around her, he said, "Sandy works until noon, of course she'd be here."

"You were kissing her!"

"Yes, I was, Mom. I happen to think a great deal of Sandy. Like I told you once before, she's the best thing to happen to Vansville." Looking his mother in the eye, he added, "She's the best thing to ever happen to me!"

Looking from him to Sandy, Millie raised her hands, but then said, "You can't..." She stopped, the words she wanted to say, dying on her lips.

Letting his hands drop from around Sandy, he straightened up and walked around his desk to his mom. Looking down at her, with steel in his eyes and an angry expression on his face, he said, "I can't what, Mom?"

With barely any breath behind the words, she murmured, "You can't kiss her! She's a cripple! You can't...." The look in his eyes stopped her cold.

Ramon's hands landed on his mom's shoulders with such force her knees buckled a little. His eyes nearly drilled holes in her. "As I told you before..." he thundered, "...you are not welcome on this property ever again. Sandy is no 'cripple' she has a handicap that she lives with, but doesn't let get her down. She is the most wonderful lady I know. You, on the other hand, are a despicable woman. If I never see you again, it won't be too soon. *Get out, get off my property and **don't come back**!*"

Two tears trickled down Millie's cheeks. That in itself was remarkable, because some of her mascara mixed with the tears and tracked down her cheeks, too. "Your own mother?" she whispered, "You'd throw me out?"

"Yes! Gladly!" He whipped her around, leaned over and pulled open the door. He nearly pushed her out through the opening, but didn't. The instant Millie cleared the door, Ramon slammed it behind her.

Sandy sat behind the desk, stunned and immobile. Other than their talking, it was quiet in the room and she could hear every word, even those Millie said in a whisper. She hadn't realized it before, but she was putting a wedge between mother and son. She couldn't do that! Ramon needed to stay in contact with his mom so he could tell her about his new faith and hopefully bring her to Christ. How could he do that if she was never allowed to come back? Even though their kisses had felt so right, she knew now that they had to be wrong.

Once Ramon slammed the door he gave it a sound kick for good measure. He moved to the desk, his chest heaving, but he didn't look at Sandy. Instead, he grabbed up the glasses and as he headed for the kitchen, he muttered, "She always makes me angry, but this time, she's gone beyond that. I'm furious!"

Ramon stalked through the door into the long hallway. For a change, he left that door open afraid he'd slam it if he touched it. Sandy wouldn't watch him. Her throat was tight and she could feel the tears burning her eyes. She looked down at the papers on the desk, they were notes from the answering machine messages, but the words were swimming before her eyes, she couldn't read them. Quickly, she pulled her sleeve across her eyes to blot them. She couldn't let her tears fall they shouldn't blur her notes to Ramon. She hadn't thought about his mom until this moment. What a rock and a hard place!

When Ramon had himself a little bit more under control, he filled the glasses with ice cubes and poured tea over them. He returned the pitcher to the refrigerator then headed back down the hall with the glasses. He set both glasses on the desk, but Sandy wouldn't look at them or him. She continued to look at the papers on the desk. How could it happen? She always tried to be so careful, but she'd forced a wedge between a son and his mother.

Ramon watched her and thought he saw her shoulders move, but he didn't hear any sound. He put his finger under her chin and raised her face, that's when he saw the tears pooled in her eyes. "Why are you crying, Sandy?" he asked kindly.

"You... you threw her out," she whispered.

"Yes, I did. I threw her out before, too, but she came back."

"She's your mom!"

He sat down in the chair beside her and nodded. "Yes, so she is. I could wish that wasn't so. I have regretted it for a very long time."

Sandy shook her head. "But Ramon, we shouldn't have kissed, it's put a barrier between you and your mom. You need to stay close so you can share your faith with her. I'm sure if she was a Christian her whole outlook would change. I'm being a wedge between you two."

Unable to understand how she could be so forgiving, he stood up and put his arm around her, making sure he continued to look into her eyes. "Sandy, she called you a 'cripple'! She's called you that before, that's why I threw her out before. That's why Isabel threw her off her property, too. I can't stand for her or anyone else to call you that! I hate that word!"

She laid her hand gently on his arm and looked up into his eyes. "But Ramon, that's what I am. I've been one all my life."

He shook his head vehemently and said, "No! You. Are. Not. A. Cripple! You have a handicap, you're paralyzed below your waist, but you aren't a cripple! That word holds such a stigma it's awful to use it about anyone. She meant it in a disparaging way she has every time she speaks of you. If there comes a time when she apologizes I might consider something different. No, Sweetheart, you are not a 'cripple', I will never think of you that way, nor allow anyone to call you that in my presence."

"Thank you, Ramon," she murmured.

"Sweetheart, there is no reason to thank me! You are a beautiful woman both on the outside but very much shining through from the inside."

Derek had fixed the Jag right after Millie's accident and brought it home. It looked brand new, better than before her accident. When it was in the garage, he told Millie that she'd either drive the fixed car or go without. He was tired of her tantrums and her finicky ways and he told her that. They lived out of town and Ramon's house was a mile from their place. She hadn't seen her son since her accident, so she reluctantly took the keys and driven to his house. When she found herself on the wrong side of the door, she hurried back to the car and fell into the driver's seat. Even before inserting the key, she grabbed her purse and fished out a tissue. Before her tears fell on her white slacks, she closed her eyes and soaked up the dampness.

Tears clogging her throat, she whimpered, "He kissed her! My son, my perfect son kissed a cripple! How could he do this to me!"

She dabbed at her eyes once more then turned the rearview mirror so she could look in it. She shook her head she must go home and fix her face before she did anything else. She pushed the mirror away she couldn't stand to look at herself with such awful smudges on her face. She inserted the key into the slot, started the car and made a wide circle in the parking lot. She almost hit Sandy's car, but stopped and backed up just in time. Tears welled up in her eyes again, but she grabbed the tissue and blotted them so they didn't slide down her cheeks.

As she drove toward her home, she wondered how she could go to the concert tonight. Derek said he was looking forward to it and she always went with him to concerts. She didn't want to go and see the awful woman who had put her claws into her son. He was supposed to marry, to give her grandchildren, but a cripple? She couldn't tolerate such a horrible thought! She drove up the drive and nearly hit the garage door before she remembered to push the opener.

Sandy watched the clock and escaped at noon. She hurried to her van and put herself inside as quickly as she could. It was good of Ramon to defend her so staunchly, but still, kissing him was wrong. They hadn't made arrangements to meet tonight, even though they both knew parking would be at a premium. The church people only parked along the streets on Sunday and none of the businesses in town had off street parking. Really, Ramon should come to her place and ride with her, but that would put them alone for a while and that might bring another kiss. She wanted another, but she knew she mustn't. She must make sure they were never alone together again. Just the thought made her heart feel like a knife was slicing it up.

When Sandy left her van and wheeled up to her front door, she saw a letter sticking out of her mailbox. She reached for it and when she recognized her dad's handwriting, she smiled. The first genuine smile since Millie came barging into Ramon's office. She hurried inside and closed the door. The envelope was fat it wasn't one sheet of paper. She wheeled herself to the kitchen and poured herself some tea, then pulled up to the table and opened her letter.

"My darling Sandy,

"I bet you're surprised to hear from your papa, aren't you? Mama usually does the writing for the family, but I felt like writing as well. Are you really doing all right? Mama seems to have this fear that something is happening with you and this man who you are working for. I keep telling her everything is fine, but I guess I need to know for myself..."

Sandy's eyes blurred and she sniffed. "Oh, Daddy," she murmured, "I don't know, I have feelings in my heart for Ramon like I have never had in all my life before for anyone. Is it right for me to have these feelings? I don't know. Maybe Mom's fears are valid, maybe something is happening between Ramon and me that shouldn't be." Her voice became only air around the words, "But it seems so right."

She finished the letter, then set it on the table and drank her iced tea. She looked at the clock and decided she'd write back to him. Her stomach was in knots, not so much from his letter, but from the events of the morning, so she didn't feel like eating. She found one of the programs for tonight's concert and decided to use the white space inside to write her letter. She'd use another sheet if she needed to.

"My precious Daddy,

"Thank you so much for writing. I'll cherish your letter for a long time. Daddy, will you keep this part of my letter to yourself for a while? It's all so new to me, but I feel I need to tell someone. Ramon came over last evening after being gone on a trail since last Saturday. A friend of his from the trail led him to the Lord. We sat and talked for a while, but then he kissed me, in fact, several times. He is a wonderful man! I have never felt for anyone as I do toward him. Is it wrong for me to feel this way? Should I try to discourage him?

Daddy, his mom doesn't like me she calls me a 'cripple' all the time. She saw us kiss at his office today and it made her furious. Ramon threw her off his property because she called me a cripple and told him he mustn't kiss me. Daddy, I don't know what to do! He just became a Believer the other day. I told him he should keep things open with his mom so he can lead her to the Lord. I wouldn't let him kiss me just before I left work, even though he tried. Daddy, what do I do...?"

She finished her letter and reread it several times, especially the first few paragraphs, hoping she said what was on her heart. Finally, she put it in an envelope. Instead of sending it to her parents' home, she addressed it to him at the post office where he worked. She was sure if it went to the house, her mom would open it and read it and if she waited for her dad to come home, she'd sit there, anxious to hear every word, because it was from her. She didn't want that to happen. As she went to the door to put the letter in the box, she looked up at her clock again and realized she had spent all afternoon agonizing over it. She still wasn't hungry, but she knew she must start to get ready for the concert.

She went inside and locked her door, then went to her closet and rummaged through her clothes, trying to decide what to wear. This was a tiny town and as Roger said, most of the people listened to bluegrass and Southern gospel, but she was playing a mostly classical concert. Mr. Casbah was coming, concerts he went to were black tie affairs and the musicians dressed in modified tuxedoes. She didn't have such a thing, but she guessed she'd better wear the next best thing. She pulled out a long black skirt that she rarely wore and a silk, long sleeved white blouse. That would have to do. With clean under clothes on her lap, she wheeled herself into the bathroom and closed the door, then maneuvered herself from her chair to the bench to take her shower. She felt the butterflies battering their wings in her stomach.

Ramon watched Sandy escape. That was the only word for it. She'd hardly said a word once she'd told him he needed to keep the lines open with his mom. He had no intention of doing that unless she went to Sandy and apologized. No, Sandy wasn't putting a wedge between himself and his mom, Millie had put the wedge there long ago. However, he knew he couldn't convince Sandy of that, maybe not ever. He shook his head. Never had such a good thing come into his life as the day that Sandy let herself down from her van and entered his office.

He sighed he had things to do for the hike the next day, so he turned from the window and headed down the hall toward his laundry room where he also kept his camping supplies and gear. Duncan was coming and he'd tentatively decided to take this group on some different trails because they'd checked them out on his computer. As he'd told Duncan, this was a church group. He wondered if they'd have a pastor with them and if they'd have devotions.

FOURTEEN

After packing his backpack the usual way and tying on his one-man tent, he took his rig to the office and set it by the door – it was ready for in the morning. From his desk drawer, he pulled out the papers Duncan had printed for him about the new area and sat down to study them. He couldn't believe it when he raised his head and stared at the clock, time had passed he must get ready for the concert.

He went to his room and looked at the clothes hanging in his closet. His step-dad and mom were coming. They often went to concerts in Atlanta and those he knew were black tie affairs. Should he dress up? He was the MC after all. He hadn't really thought about it, but maybe he should, maybe even a string tie would be appropriate. He went in his attached bathroom to take a shower and wash his hair. He would look his best for Sandy even if no one else appreciated it. She was every reason to dress in his best clothes, not to impress her, but to show how much she meant to him.

He sighed after his shower as he dressed. He'd wanted to go with her, to ride in her van with her and walk in with her. In fact, he wanted to spend all the time he could with her. After how she'd fled the office this noon, he wasn't sure what to do. He pulled on his black slacks and tucked his black silk shirt into them. If he wanted that to happen, he'd better get to her place just after six. He knew she planned to be at the church by six thirty. He was sure she wanted to go over things, just once more. He looked at his watch, it was nearly time and he hadn't eaten.

Ramon grabbed two granola bars and left. After he had his truck in gear, he ripped open the first bar and bit off a huge bite. On the road, he chewed furiously and popped the rest of the bar into his mouth as he wheeled onto Isabel's parking lot. He pulled behind Sandy's van as Isabel walked out of her house and Sandy wheeled herself down her walk toward her van.

Ramon took one long look and his breath clogged his throat, he couldn't seem to suck in any air. He'd never seen her so beautiful. The white blouse she had on sparkled in the long rays of the setting sun. Her hair glistened and she had tiny dangling earrings that also sparkled on her earlobes. He couldn't take his eyes from her, but she didn't seem to notice him, just wheeled herself to the back of the van and inserted the key to open the door.

"Ramon!" Isabel called. "You're in time! I'm glad you came to ride with us, I'm sure parking will be bad. Can you imagine in our little town?"

He chuckled at that. "Yeah, Isabel, it might even come down to a traffic jam! By the way, Isabel, you look really nice this evening."

"Why, thank you, Sonny!"

Sandy was still on the ground, but wheeling herself on the lift when he walked up. Before she could hit the control for the lift, he stepped onto it with her. Surprised, she looked up at him and he smiled down at her. For her ears alone, he said, "You, Sweetheart, take my breath away. You are totally lovely this evening."

She forgot to push the button for several seconds, so they were still on the ground when Isabel walked up. "Missy, aren't you going to raise that thing?"

Feeling really foolish and feeling the heat rise on her neck, she finally swallowed and said, "Oh, yes, of course, Isabel. I was thinking how handsome Ramon looks. He'll be a real hit as the MC. Don't you think?"

Looking the young man up and down, Isabel said, "Sure enough! Ramon, will you send that lift back down so I can ride it and sit on that back bench?"

"Of course, Isabel."

Sandy opened her mouth to protest, she wasn't sure what. She wanted Ramon to sit up front with her, but Isabel was an old lady, she shouldn't sit on that back bench, it was much harder than the front seat where she usually sat. Isabel winked at Ramon and he grinned back at her. He was pretty sure she knew both his and Sandy's feelings. Sandy didn't say anything, she finally closed her mouth and pushed the button so she and Ramon could enter the van, then Ramon sent it back down for Isabel.

Isabel happily sat on the bench and Ramon slithered into the passenger seat, while Sandy fastened her chair behind the wheel. Ramon wondered briefly why Sandy had no music, but then he realized the last time he'd come while she was playing she'd had no music in front of her. She must have the whole program memorized. Not that his opinion of her was low to start with, but his esteem for her went up another notch.

Roger had told Sandy there would be a ramp for her to use, but she hadn't seen it, since the church was at the other end of town from her cabin. Ramon hadn't seen it either, but he didn't know there was to be one. It was before six thirty, but already there were several cars parked in front of the church and across the street in front of the hardware store. Sandy maneuvered her van into a space that was barely big enough, but into a position where she could lower the lift and get out on the sidewalk, only a little ways from the ramp.

"Wow! When did that pile of wood arrive?" Ramon asked, peering out the windshield.

"Roger got his church men to put it up this week so Sandy could get in. All there were before were those five steps. I came for some gas the other day and saw him down on his knees painting those boards. He oughtta get down on his knees for another reason, to my way of thinkin'." Isabel said, as Sandy put the van in park. Sandy nodded in agreement, but didn't say anything as she reached for the lift controls.

The man in question came from the church and took the five steps in two. Ramon looked at him he was dressed the same way he'd dressed when Ramon had come to the church to ask about a concert. Of course, Roger didn't have anything to do with the program, he didn't have to be on the platform, but Roger didn't look like he was doing more than going to a movie with his buddies. Ramon felt embarrassed for Sandy.

Sandy hadn't said a word on the way. She also held her comment, if she'd planned to say anything, about Roger's attire. As soon as Sandy shut off the van, Isabel was on her feet and pushed the button so that the door opened. Ramon hadn't even left the passenger seat and Sandy hadn't released her chair from behind the steering wheel before Isabel was on the ground.

She looked Roger up and down and said, "Sonny, don't you have anything better to wear to the first concert we've ever had in this town?"

She didn't see him swallow or his Adam's apple bounce, she was sending the lift back up for Ramon and Sandy. "Yes, Ma'am," he finally said.

"Well, you got time you go home and get it on! Why, the idea of the preacher looking like a tramp when a concert's being held in his church!"

"Yes, Ma'am. I'll just do that!"

Sandy lowered her head, but Ramon could see the grin on her face. He looked at her, his eyes twinkling. Sandy looked up to see Roger running away from them to his Jeep. Softly, she said, "I guess she told him."

Ramon couldn't hold it in any longer, his laughter bubbled up from his chest. "Yup, I guess she did. Look at him run!"

She backed out from behind the steering wheel just as Ramon stood up. She reached for his hand and he grasped it. "Thanks for coming to the cabin, even though we didn't talk about it. You really look spectacular in that outfit."

"Sandy, not near what you do! This evening you are the most beautiful woman in all the world! I'm proud to be with you."

"Stop it! I can't cry!" she said, breathless.

"Why? Will your makeup run?" Sandy only nodded.

"Mommie," a tiny voice whispered, "isn't that 'Twinkle, Twinkle, Little Star'? How come she's playin' that?"

The lady put her lips right beside the child's ear and whispered, "I guess she wanted to play something you'd know."

A grin broke across the little girl's face and she clapped her hands. "Oh, yes!"

There was one other piece that many of the people were familiar with, but most of the audience was in awe of the lady who made the ivories sing. Sandy lost herself in the music it was nothing like the last time she'd played a concert. Then it had been in her home church, she'd known most of the people. She'd grown up knowing most of those who came to hear her play, they all thought of her as 'poor little Sandy', they'd come out of sympathy, not because of her talent, but tonight, she only knew a few of those who came, so she had no preconceptions to over come at all. The place was packed in fact there was standing room only. Roger was one of those standing in the back. Derek and Millie were there, sitting in a very prominent seat.

The instant she raised her hands from the last piece before the intermission the applause was thunderous. However, she nearly ripped off the black pouch from her chair then disappeared behind the door beside the platform and Ramon joined her. He walked in right behind her, kicked the door closed and didn't stop until he had his arms around her and was kissing her soundly. "You are magnificent! Sandy, your performance has been awesome!" he said, when they came up for air.

She smiled, but all she said was, "Thanks."

They stayed there in the little room the entire fifteen minutes Sandy didn't want to be talking to anyone before she played the last and hardest piece. She knew it all perfectly, but parts of it were very intricate and she felt she needed to visualize it in her mind before her fingers rested on the keys.

When fifteen minutes were over, Roger came to the door, opened it only a few inches, just enough to stick his head in and say, "You're on, the lights are down."

Ramon followed Sandy out, she stopped at the piano and Ramon climbed the stairs to the platform. He looked out at the audience; there was not an empty seat in the place. The whole village had come to hear the very first concert ever given in the little town and many from Isabel's church in Blairsville came because she'd asked them.

Ramon smiled and said, "Ladies and gentlemen, Sandy and I want to thank you for being such a good audience. She will now play her final number on the program."

Because it was such a long piece, Sandy had suggested he leave the platform and sit down close by while she played, so she waited until he was seated. There was no sound in the room as Sandy raised her hands and silently placed them on the keyboard. It was a dramatic first chord and Sandy played it accordingly, but then her fingers flew across the keys. All eyes were glued to her as she played. Everyone was enthralled, Ramon being one of them. He wasn't sure, but he wondered if Mr. Chopin himself could have played any better.

When she lifted her hands, there was a momentary silence, but then Derek Casbah jumped to his feet, yelling, "Bravo, Bravo!" and clapped loudly.

Only seconds later, everyone was on his feet clapping. Ramon clapped as he made his way to the platform Sandy had done a magnificent job. Ramon stood at the podium, waiting for the clapping and cheers to quiet, but before he could speak, Derek called out, "Encore, encore!" Others quickly took up the chant.

Ramon stopped clapping, stepped to the podium and raised his hand. When the place quieted so he could be heard, he smiled and said, "Ms Bernard has a favorite piece she'd like to play for you folks. She has asked me to tell you that this arrangement is her own work. She composed it for her former students in Philadelphia. Enjoy."

Everyone sat quickly and Ramon stepped back from the podium and sat on the platform. Again, Sandy began to play. This one was a favorite of hers; her own composition using nursery rhymes that had been set to music. She started each one with one finger playing the melody then when she'd played it through once she'd start her own variation. Soon, one little voice, then another began to sing with her. Sandy smiled and joined in as she played the familiar tunes.

This time, when she finished the piece the hand clapping sounded different. The first ones to clap were the children. Although the adults soon joined, it was the children who yelled their praise. Sandy slid the black pouch from her chair, then backed away from the piano and turned around, soon the children crowded around her chair, most of them talking and hugging her. To anyone watching, it was obvious how much she loved children. Several of her friends wondered if she could have any of her own. Isabel sat watching and shaking her head, a tear slid down her cheek. The girl was awesome!

Only a few minutes later the parents began coming to collect their children and each one said how much they enjoyed her concert. Ramon stood with her, not to receive any praise, but because he wanted to. After the children were gone with their parents, the adults who were in the audience came to shake hands and give their words of praise. It would be an understatement to say that Sandy was overwhelmed. Ramon could see it in her eyes.

Almost everyone had left when Derek Casbah came up with his hand out. "Ms. Bernard, I have never enjoyed a concert more than what you played tonight. That last piece on the program you played like the master himself. In fact, I have a recording of that very piece and you played it as well or better than is played on that recording. Thank you for a very enjoyable evening. I truly hope you will do this again."

Sandy took his hand and shook it warmly. "Why, Mr. Casbah, thank you! Thank you so much! I really appreciate your kind words. I also want to thank you for getting this piano tuned for tonight. I hadn't played on it before, so I don't know how out-of-tune it was, but it was a joy to play this evening."

Derek shuddered and made a face. He held her hand, caressing it just a little. "I asked around town. No one who's lived her a long time knew how long it had been since it was tuned last, so it absolutely had to be done. I cannot abide an out-of-tune piano, especially for a piano concert." He still held Sandy's hand and as he looked at her intently, he said, "You will play another concert for us soon, won't you?"

Sandy laughed, her eyes twinkling. "When you put it that way, it doesn't seem like I have too much choice, does it?"

Derek also smiled. "Good!" He dropped Sandy's hand, turned and stepped back. "I'll be waiting for the announcement." Shaking his finger at her he added, "Young lady, that announcement better not be too long in coming!"

Millie had been standing behind her husband looking very uncomfortable. Derek had said all he wanted to say, so as he turned away it left a clear path from Sandy and Ramon to Millie. Both Sandy and Ramon felt it was Millie's obligation to speak first, but their faces were very different. Sandy's was open and she was smiling at Millie, Ramon was scowling at his mom with no sign of friendliness. He wanted to usher her out, but he didn't move.

Tentatively, very hesitantly, Millie stepped forward and held out her hand to Sandy. She never raised her eyes to her son, but she looked at Sandy and said, "You were very good. I was impressed with everything you did." Before Sandy could speak, Millie rushed on, "Could I commission you to paint a picture?"

The smile encompassing her face, Sandy reached for the woman's hand to shake and said, "Certainly, Mrs. Casbah, do you have something in mind? By the way, thank you for your compliment, I appreciate that."

"Actually, what I have in mind is something quite large. You see, I have a place over the fireplace in my great room that could hold something as large as those four pictures you have hanging in Ramon's office. It is a panorama, isn't it?"

"Yes. You'd like something like that?"

Nodding, she said, "Something as wide as those four put together, and… and maybe square, you know?"

"Those four can be hung side by side to look like one picture or I can special order a canvas about that size. It's up to you, Mrs. Casbah. What scene would you like and what season of the year did you have in mind?"

Millie sighed then looked around the auditorium. "In a few weeks the fall colors will be at their best. My great room takes its color scheme from the sandstone rocks of the fireplace. That means they're earthtones, making the room rather dark. Miss Bernard, if you made your picture with those fall colors in it I would like that very much."

"All right, I'll wait a few weeks and take some pictures, then let you choose which scene you'd like to have. Oh, by the way, I'd like you to call me Sandy."

Millie smiled a tiny smile for the first time. "Thank you. Actually, could I take the picture and give it to you?"

"Of course, that would be perfect. However, I'll go ahead and order a large canvas so I'll have it ready when you have the picture."

"Thanks, I'll mail it to you," she whispered.

Finally, Millie looked up at her son, who had lost his scowl, but who'd just snapped his mouth closed. What his mom had done had him totally baffled. "You were right. This lady is the best thing to happen to Vansville in a very long time."

Nodding, Ramon said, "I totally agree, Mom."

Millie looked around and realized that Derek stood at the back of the church chatting with Roger, but waiting for her to join him. Isabel had gone outside, so there were only five of them still left in the building. Millie smiled tentatively at both of the young people and said, "I guess my husband's waiting for me, but I did want to ask you about that. Thank you again. I'll be in touch."

"Yes, Mrs. Casbah."

Sandy turned back to the piano. She had taken the black pouch off of her chair as soon as she finished playing, but not disconnected it from the piano. Now that everyone had left she must work with the wires from her pouch that she'd hooked to the piano when she came. It wasn't hard, but she did have to be careful. The wires could break easily.

When his mom was at the back door, Ramon muttered, "I can't believe that! I guess she's finally decided to take both Isabel and me seriously. She'll mail you her picture. Wow!"

Sandy took the little pouch from where she'd laid it on the piano keys and handed it to Ramon to hold while she unhooked the wires from the piano. "Yes, I think she has, but I think she wishes she could still come see you."

He shook his head as he gave the pouch back to her. "She'll have to do lots more than that to get back on my property, believe me!"

Sandy laid the pouch on her lap and Ramon walked beside her as she wheeled herself down the main aisle toward the door. Sandy was beginning to feel the effects of ninety minutes of playing, but it was a good feeling. By the time they reached the foyer, Derek and Millie had left and only Roger still stood inside. He reached for the switch to turn out the lights at the front of the church. He flashed a grin at the couple as the lights clicked off, leaving them in the much more intimate light of the tiny foyer. Since he'd gone home to change, he looked exceptionally handsome, but the man beside Sandy sent her heart into fits, while the man in front of her did nothing to her heart at all. This flutter in her heart was an amazing phenomenon no one in all her life had ever sent her heart into flutters. Really, she had no idea what the sensation meant.

Roger reached for Sandy's hand and shook it. "I would say that you were the biggest hit this town has ever had. You played magnificently tonight, Sandy."

Sandy smiled and shook his hand. "Thank you, Roger. I enjoyed doing it, much more than the last concert I gave."

He chuckled. "If I'd have been a preaching kind of man I might have been tempted to get up and sermonize to such a full house."

Sandy knew he was joking, but she intended to use every chance to win this man to the Lord, she smiled, hoping her next words were palatable, "Roger, you give them the Word and you just might have to punch out a wall. Thanks for letting us use your building tonight."

"Yeah, sure," he said with much less enthusiasm.

Sandy turned from Roger and headed for the door. Ramon opened it and as she crossed the threshold, she said, "Roger, tell whoever put up this ramp that I appreciate it immensely. At that other concert I played, even though it was in my home church, they'd never thought it necessary to put up a ramp for my use, even though I was there every week for services. For my concert, my dad had to carry me in and back out, while my brother bounced my chair up, then down the steps."

"Oh, my!" Ramon and Roger said together. "You were an adult?" Roger added.

"Almost, I was eighteen."

"Unbelievable!" Ramon exclaimed.

Isabel stood on the sidewalk chatting with some friends and waiting for Sandy and Ramon to come out. It was dark, the only light came from the light in the entryway of the church and a streetlight in front of Brad's store across the street. Roger turned out the rest of the lights then stood in the doorway watching as Sandy wheeled herself down the ramp with Ramon right beside her. He sighed it was even more obvious tonight that Ramon had staked his claim on the beautiful Sandy Bernard.

Oblivious to Roger and his thoughts, Sandy wheeled herself to the van. Now there were hardly any parked cars along the street and as the lady talking with Isabel saw Sandy, she moved away toward her own car. Sandy smiled at the lady, but she was ready to call this evening to a close, so she went to the back of the van and opened the large door. As soon as the lift was on the sidewalk, Isabel said a hasty farewell to her friend and scrambled on and hit the button to take her up, then she sent it back for Sandy and Ramon.

When they were on, Isabel sat on the back seat already and Sandy sighed, "Isabel, that is a hard seat, I've used it as a bed. You should sit up front."

"Missy, that seat is for your beau. Now don't you argue with me, just get up there and drive us home. It's almost my bedtime."

Sandy sighed again, but she heard Ramon chuckle softly, as he headed for the passenger seat. Without another word, she wheeled herself into the driver's position and locked her chair in place. She took a moment and pulled in a deep breath, then started up, turned around in the gas station lot and headed back down Main Street toward Isabel's cabins.

When they were on the street, Isabel said, "Missy, I'm so glad we had this concert! It was wonderful and now everybody in town knows what a few of us already knew, that you are one exceptional lady."

"I'll second that!" Ramon said, enthusiastically.

"Thank you, both of you," Sandy said, as she turned the wheel onto Isabel's gravel parking lot.

As soon as Sandy had the van in place, Isabel was on her way out. From the ground, she said, "I'll see you both another day." She hurried to her house and had the door closed and the porch light off before Sandy had the van locked up.

Sandy shook her head. "That lady is something else!" She looked up at Ramon in the light of the one streetlight and said, "You know, I think that lady's matchmaking."

Ramon chuckled and stepped up beside Sandy so he could put his hand on the back of her neck. "Sweetheart, I'm pretty sure you're right, but you know, it doesn't bother me at all, if you must know the truth."

Ramon's hand on her neck sent a shiver down Sandy's spine. She couldn't feel it below her waist, but she was sure it went all the way to her toes. This man did things to her that she'd never experienced before. "But Ramon," she exclaimed, "you haven't made peace with your mom! She talked nicely to me tonight and I'm glad, but you haven't built a bridge with her. You need to, you need to show her your new love for Christ and let her know she needs Him."

"Give it time, Sweetheart, maybe it'll happen. I noticed you left Roger less than enthusiastic there at the back of the church."

While she inserted the key into her door, she said very seriously, "Ramon, there is a verse in Scripture that says that a man who calls himself a teacher or leader of people has more responsibility and more punishment if he leads people astray. That is the situation Roger would find himself in at the judgment. It truly is a serious place to be for one who stands in front of a gathering in a church every seven days."

Ramon whistled as he walked in behind Sandy.

She smiled at him and asked, "Would you like some iced tea?"

Ramon looked at her and said, "I'll get it. You go sit on the couch. You've done all the work tonight and I can surely fill two glasses with ice and tea. Ever since I saw you coming out your door before the concert I wanted to kiss you and hold you on my lap. It's gonna happen as soon as I get back with that tea."

With a huge grin on her face, she gave him a two finger salute and said, "Aye, aye, Sir. I'm on my way!"

When he came from the kitchen with two glasses, Sandy was sitting close to one end of the couch and her chair was abandoned a few feet away. Ramon set the glasses down on the coffee table close by, scooped her up as if she were a feather and sat down where she had been sitting. He barely had her on his lap when his lips claimed hers. Their tea sat forgotten, the ice melting until the top inch was hardly colored at all.

When Ramon finally laid his forehead on hers, he said, in a ragged voice, "You know, that must last until Wednesday night."

"Will you get back before supper?"

"I plan to, Sweetheart."

"It'll be waiting for you here."

He looked up at the clock and sighed. "One more kiss then I must go. I think Duncan will be here before the rest and I plan to take them on an all new trail this time."

"Ramon, do be careful!"

"I'll do my best. I take every precaution I possibly can. You know I made that special trip to buy a cell phone, too. From now on that'll be standard equipment. I made sure I could keep it charged and usable on any hike of any length."

Renewing her hold on his neck, she kissed him and said, "I know you do, but I still think about you and pray for you while you're gone."

"Thanks, I'm glad for that."

Ramon had hardly closed the door behind him when Sandy's phone rang. Since she was not in her chair, she was glad for the extension she'd hooked up beside the couch, so she reached for it. Her parents knew she was to play a concert tonight, perhaps it was them. "Hello?" she said, as Ramon's truck started up outside.

"Hello, my dear. How did your concert go?"

"Daddy! It was wonderful! It was nothing like the one when I played there at your church. Daddy, one of those who came goes to concerts regularly in Atlanta. When I finished, he jumped to his feet yelling 'Bravo, Bravo!' I couldn't believe it. The place was packed they even filled the aisles with extra chairs. Everyone came up to me and told me what a wonderful time they had. I only got home a few minutes ago."

"Sandy, I'm so pleased! Did you get any pupils from it?"

"Daddy, I never thought to ask, but my encore was my Variations on Nursery Rhymes and the children flocked around after that. Perhaps I'll get some calls another day. Ramon's step-dad asked if I would play soon again, made it almost mandatory. Much to everyone's surprise, he employed a piano tuner to tune it this morning. That made it sound even better. Ramon had a falling out with his mom, but she asked me to paint her a large panorama for her great room wall. I'm so busy, Daddy, I fall into bed and sleep straight through to morning."

"I'm so glad to hear that, Honey."

"Sandy, are you sure you're doing all right? No one is hurting you?"

"Hi, Mom, no everyone is very nice. For a while Ramon's mom was quite antagonistic, but now that she's commissioned me to paint for her, I think that's over."

"I wanted to come down and see you, but your dad and brother talked me out of it, so we haven't come. You will be home for Christmas, didn't you say?" Charlie cleared his throat, but didn't say anything. All three of them knew that was not exactly what Colleen had wanted to do, but he wouldn't correct her.

Remembering Ramon's kisses and how wonderful it felt to sit in his arms a few minutes ago, Sandy realized she didn't want to leave him for any amount of time at all, especially all the way to Philadelphia. She wanted to be here. It had become really hard to have him go off on a trail, and that was close by, not hundreds of miles away.

Finally she said, "Mom, Christmas is several months away. Yes, I'd planned to come home then, but we'll have to see how things are working here. Ramon only asked me yesterday if I'd help him over the winter to get things organized for the new season next spring. With piano projects and painting, I think I'll be busy, but like I said, we'll see how things work out. At this point it's hard to tell."

Colleen's voice was almost a wail, as she said, "Sandy! You must come home! It's not right for you to stay gone so long!"

"Mom?"

Sandy waited in the silence until Colleen whispered, "Yes?"

She knew everyone in her family had said almost these exact words before, but she said, "Mom, Daddy left Germany nearly thirty years ago, he's never been back. I don't intend to stay away for thirty years, but things here have changed since I talked with you about coming home. Keep that in mind, okay?"

Colleen's voice broke as she said, "Sandy, you must come home!"

"Mom, it's good to talk with you, I'll see you sometime. Bye, Daddy, I love you."

"Goodbye, my dear. I'm glad the concert was such a success."

Sandy hung up quickly she didn't want to have her mom spoil her evening.

Charlie heard the click of Sandy's phone, so he hung up too, but Colleen sat beside him still holding the cordless phone to her ear. Slowly she pulled it down from her face, but didn't disconnect it. Charlie looked at her and realized she was crying. Big, silent tears were sliding down her cheeks. He wondered how much longer Colleen would try to hold a torch for Sandy, surely not her whole life! One of these days she must understand that Sandy was not coming home to live ever again and if he could read the signs very well, she would be getting married before another summer came around.

"Mama," he asked, as he took the phone from her and pushed the disconnect button. "What is it? Why are you crying?"

"She won't come home on her own! What'll happen before Christmas? I can't stand this house without her. We must go get her before she looses her heart to that place. I knew that concert was a bad idea." Colleen sniffled and shook her head. "Charlie, when can we go?"

Charlie waited for Colleen to look at him. Her tears kept falling there was a long silence before she finally looked at him. Even though she continued to cry, she sniffed and finally gave him her undivided attention. He said, "Mama, it was *not* a bad idea! I'm glad she was able to perform. That time she played at our church was awful for her. Those people made her feel like a sad little peasant girl on the corner wanting alms!"

Devastated, Colleen wept, "But didn't you hear? Every other word was something about Ramon! We must get her home before something dreadful happens to her. Don't you see?"

"Colleen, look at me!" Charlie waited until Colleen raised her head again and turned it toward him. Tears still hung on her lashes, but he could tell she would listen. "Listen to me very carefully." He continued to look into her eyes. "Colleen, Sandy is a grown woman.

Young women have desires, wishes and ambitions. Our eldest has them, just as you had them as a young woman before we met. If she meets a young man who will love her and cherish her as his wife, will you be a wedge between them?"

"I want what's best for my daughter!" Before Charlie could speak, Colleen hurried on, "What's best for her is to be here at home! How can you say some man can love and cherish her?" Colleen shook her head. "No, it can't...."

Charlie took her hand and said, tenderly, "Colleen, have you prayed about this? Has the Lord told you that Sandy must be here, living with us?"

Colleen dropped her head, but Charlie saw her shake her head, while she whispered, "But it's best, it has to be!"

Quietly, but very emphatically, Charlie said, "No, my love, if the Lord wants to fulfill her life with a loving, Christian young man, then that's what's best. Mama, do you remember when Sandy was a baby how we took her to church and gave her to the Lord?"

After a long silence, she whispered, "I remember."

Stroking her arm and tenderly kissing her, he whispered into her ear, "I wondered. Are you taking that gift back now that she's twenty-five?"

Colleen's tears flowed down her cheeks again. "I want to."

"I know that, but you may not, my love." Charlie took a deep breath and said, "Sandy decided to move to north Georgia and she is making her life there."

"I wish she'd never seen that add in that magazine," she mumbled.

"But she did."

Just as he'd suspected, Duncan arrived as Ramon poured his coffee. When he heard the SUV on the parking lot, he pulled another mug from the cupboard and poured more coffee. He'd already scrambled some eggs in his bowl, so he took several more from the refrigerator and broke them into the same bowl. When Ramon heard the knock on his door, he had the golden liquid sizzling in his frying pan. He popped two pieces of bread in the toaster.

"Come on in, Duncan! I figured you'd get here early."

The blond giant pushed the door open, walked across the living room to the kitchen. Grinning he said, "I hoped I'd get here for eats. Even a cup of coffee ready to drink! Thanks."

Still stirring the eggs, Ramon asked, "Would you fix the toast? I have the bread right beside the toaster. The first slices should be up in a second."

"Sure! Wasn't that some concert? Except to see it with my own eyes, I wouldn't have believed it possible for her to play so well. That little black pouch on her chair is part of it?"

Nodding, Ramon said, "I knew she was good before, but she beat it all. Yes, she uses her shoulder on that pouch to work the sustaining pedal."

Duncan pulled out the bread from the wrapper, put it in the toaster slots and pushed the lever down. He picked up his mug and took a long sip, then turned to look at Ramon as he flipped the eggs around in the pan. "Are you soft on her?"

A smile touched Ramon's lips, then grew as he looked up at his new friend. "You mean do I think she's the most wonderful, beautiful, exceptional woman to come into my life since I learned about chocolate cake on my first birthday? And ice cream that I could smear into my mouth before sucking it off my hands?"

Duncan threw back his head and laughed. "I'd say I got my answer," he finally said, but immediately grew serious. "But doesn't her chair and her... her paralysis bother you?" he asked.

As Ramon scooped two large helpings of eggs onto two plates he shook his head. "I hardly even see her chair. It doesn't bother me at all. She is so full of life and so happy all the time that I rarely even think about it."

"What do her parents think about you?"

"I haven't a clue. She rarely talks about her parents. I think her mom was highly opposed to her leaving home, but her dad is very supportive of everything she does. She said her mom didn't want her piano shipped, probably as a means to get her home. Believe me, I'm still dealing with my own mom's reaction to her."

Duncan placed the plate of toast on the table then pulled out the chair Ramon motioned him to and said, "Less than cordial, I take it?"

Ramon picked up a piece of toast, then his fork and scooped up a large forkful of eggs, before he said, "Mmm, until last night when she commissioned Sandy to paint her a huge picture for over her mantel in her great room."

"That's progress."

"Possibly," Ramon said, dubiously.

They each ate their eggs and toast, but then Duncan took a long swill of coffee. Still holding the mug, he pulled the napkin from his shirt front and said, "I heard there's another tropical storm gaining momentum down by Bermuda. It could get here before this hike is over in five days. Would your hikers wimp out with that forecast?"

Ramon groaned. "The last one was horrible and sent someone to the hospital. I hope it's tuckered out before it reaches here."

Duncan nodded, picked up his plate and mug and went to the sink. He put the plate in the sink, but filled his cup with coffee. "Right, one could only hope."

Ramon followed suit and said, "Let's take our coffee to the office."

Soon after they finished eating, the hikers arrived. By now, Ramon and Duncan were going over their maps in the office, so they watched as car doors slammed and trunks popped open. Usually, seeing a group of hikers arrive worked Ramon's blood into a rush, but today he realized taking these hikers out took him away from a very special lady, one he'd love to hold in his arms every day for the rest of his life. His line of work wasn't very conducive for that.

The leader knocked then walked in the office. He looked between the two men and asked, "Is one of you Ramon?"

The young man grinned and held out his hand. "Yes, that would be me. My new associate has asked to join us. This is Duncan Roads."

The man held out his hand. "Good to meet you. I'm Bob Ways." He turned back to Ramon and said, "I told my group to wait out there, that they didn't all need to pile in here just to turn around and head out again."

Ramon chuckled, nodding. "Good. We're ready, so let's head out and get on the trail."

Nodding, the man said, "Sounds good!"

Duncan went out behind the group leader, but Ramon circled his desk and grabbed his new cell phone from the charger. If he didn't turn it on unless he needed it, the man at the store who had sold it to him assured him it would not loose its charge in a week. Ramon was counting on it. He planned never to use it except for an emergency as there was during the last hurricane they'd survived. He'd heard about the tropical storm on the news last night, but he was hoping that it would bypass them, even head into the Gulf or die a natural death off some other coast.

He clipped the phone to his belt, picked up his gear by the shoulder straps and headed out. He turned the lock on the door and pulled it closed. Sandy wasn't far from his thoughts, but he needed to focus on the new trails and the group he was leading, so he hadn't called her. He told her last night that he wouldn't see her or talk to her until he was back Wednesday afternoon.

As Ramon turned, all the people were shouldering their backpacks. "Folks," he said, "I need to ask a couple things before we head out. Are there enough tents for everyone to sleep inside and do you all have some kind of raingear?"

"Yes," Bob answered, "I made sure before we left this morning that we had enough two man tents for everyone to sleep inside and I also made sure we all had rain slickers. I'm sure you're aware of the tropical storm that's off shore."

"Yes, I'm aware of it. How's everyone's footgear? Do you all have hiking boots or something very, very similar?"

Everyone nodded and Bob again said, "Yes. We do."

FIFTEEN

Duncan was not like Ramon, of course, he wasn't the last-word leader, but that evening when they stopped to set up camp, Bob said they'd have devotions following supper. Duncan looked at Ramon and gave him a look that could only be interpreted to mean that Duncan would not be around to listen. Ramon saw himself at the beginning of the summer in his expression.

Later, as the group settled down and several pulled Bibles from their packs, Duncan wandered off into the woods. Ramon realized that other years and at first this summer he had been like that. For nearly twenty-seven years he'd turned his back on God. Actually, his mom had never given him an opportunity to learn about God. Sandy had come into his life and although she wasn't the one to lead him to Christ, she had been the one who softened his heart. He stifled a chuckle, she'd softened his heart in more ways than to the Lord, but he felt wonderful. He knew he'd never been in love before, but this feeling he had toward Sandy, he knew he was in love with her.

As the leader started with Scripture Ramon listened closely. This was a different passage than he'd heard before, but he wanted to learn all he could. He listened to Bob's remarks and bowed his head when he prayed to close the short devotional. Ramon hadn't participated, but as the leader said, "Amen," Ramon felt the peace of God wash over him. It was dark and Duncan hadn't returned as the group headed for their tents. Ramon's custom was to wait until everyone was accounted for, so he still sat by the campfire. It was a pleasant evening mosquitoes weren't bad around the fire, so Ramon was happy to sit in the quietness.

Bob still held his Bible as he came and sat down beside Ramon. After watching the fire burn lower for several minutes, Bob asked, "Ramon, are you a Christian?"

Ramon pulled one leg up and rested his arm on his knee. He turned and grinned at the older man and said, "Yes, I am! Not a very old Christian, but I am one."

Bob grinned back at Ramon and exclaimed, "Great! That's terrific! Could you tell me your experience?"

"I believe you called the other day and talked with my receptionist, Sandy?"

"Yes, she sounded like a really sweet person on the phone."

"She is! Anyway, almost as soon as she came back in August she asked me if I was a Christian. I assured her I was not and had no interest in becoming one. She told me she'd be praying for me. Well, several of the groups I've led this summer are like yours, a church group. One not long ago also had devotions in the evenings and especially two of the passages the youth pastor read worked their way into my thoughts. I couldn't banish them as I had before.

"Over Labor Day, some seasoned hikers whom I know went with Duncan and me on a rugged trail. One of those men had recently become a Christian. We talked that first night and God softened my heart and I asked Him to be my Savior the second evening."

The pastor laid his hand on Ramon's shoulder and squeezed it. "Ramon, I'm really glad to hear that! Duncan hasn't done that yet, has he?"

Ramon shook his head, watching the fire burn low. "No, he'd have nothing to do with my friend that weekend and when I told him this group was a church group, he told me you folks had better not force it down his throat. I assured him that wouldn't happen." Ramon grinned again. "I didn't tell him we wouldn't pray for him, though."

Bob chuckled. "Good for you, Ramon. We'll do that. Let's do it now." Both men bowed their heads and after a moment's silence,

Bob said, "Dear Father, I'm so glad to know that Ramon has recently become Your child, but he tells me that his associate, Duncan, wants nothing to do with You. We know that You're in the business of changing and softening people's hearts and we pray that You will with Duncan. He needs You, Lord, bring him to Yourself we pray. In Your Son's name, amen."

"Amen," Ramon added softly.

Bob left and climbed into his tent, but Ramon sat by the fire because Duncan still wasn't back. Ramon didn't fret about his absence, but he would wait for the man, besides, he enjoyed the quietness. Finally, only the stars and a warm glow in the firepit were the only light when Duncan came through the trees. He saw Ramon and hurried over. He picked up a stick and poked at the fire, bringing it back to life. Duncan flopped down and they sat for several minutes being quiet, listening to the night sounds around them.

Finally, Duncan said, "You didn't have to wait for me. You could have headed for the sack. I'm okay."

Ramon shrugged and turned his head to look at the man. "I know that, Duncan, but I always make it a practice not to bed down myself until I know everyone is in camp. These people pay good money for me to be responsible for them while we're on the trail, so I take the job seriously. I know you will when you lead your own groups, but it's a thing with me that I started with my first group."

"Thanks, Ramon, I'll remember that."

Tuesday evening, it clouded over as it had the last time a hurricane had come ashore. Then it worked its way up the coast and it was no different this time. Sandy watched the clouds move in. She sat on her porch after supper and instead of a glorious sunset, dark clouds covered the sun before it reached the horizon. Ramon had to see them, he wasn't far away. Days were getting shorter, it would be fall soon. That meant two things, Ramon wouldn't be taking groups hiking and there might be snow in this higher elevation. Sandy had never driven in snow, it was not something she was anxious to do, either, but she wouldn't let it discourage her.

During the night, the rain came. Sandy heard it pelting her window even before she opened her eyes in the morning. She shuddered, she hated to get out in the rain, no matter how she dressed she was always wet when she arrived at her destination. That's how it was, they didn't make rain slickers large enough to fit over her in a sitting position and at the same time cover her chair motor. However, as she got ready to leave, she put on her slicker, letting it cover her head and the back of her chair to keep her battery dry then she found the big piece of plastic she'd used before to cover her lap and pulled it up as far under the slicker as she could. She'd be as dry as possible when she arrived at work. As she left her home, she remembered the last time they'd had rain like this when Ramon had a group out, someone had gotten hurt and had to be airlifted out she prayed it wouldn't happen again.

There was no grove of trees to camp under when Ramon brought the group to their last campsite. He'd watched all afternoon as the clouds built in the south, then more joining them from the west. Before the group left the campfire after their devotions, Ramon said, "Folks, I'm sure it'll be raining before we get up in the morning. Be sure when you bed down that you move everything away from the sides of your tents. Anything that touches the sides draws dampness, you can be very wet if it rains much."

"We'll hike in the rain?" one girl asked.

"Of course, silly," her brother snorted his answer. "Nobody's going to come out here with a van to cart you back warm and dry. Camping is just that, you set up *camp* outside and you take whatever Mother Nature sends your way."

She glared at her brother, then she and her friends turned without comment and climbed into their tents. The boy shrugged, girls could be so stupid, but it showed the most when they were doing outdoor stuff. He and his friends also turned toward the tents.

Only a few minutes later, Duncan came back from his walk and said, "We won't be bedded down long before the rain comes. I could see it a couple of hills away."

Quickly, everyone who wasn't in his tent vanished and several zippers went down at the same time. Ramon and Duncan were the last into their tents and Ramon hadn't even stretched out when he heard the first drop hit his green roof. He pulled off his boots and slid into his sleeping bag, wishing he was home, not in his own home, but down the road in a certain cabin where a lovely lady would welcome him. His mouth already watered for whatever she planned to have for supper and that would be twenty-four hours from now.

He sighed and closed his eyes. "Lord, keep us safe in the rain tomorrow."

It was morning, but to look at the sky one could hardly tell. Ramon groaned and scrambled from his sleeping bag. As he usually did, he rolled his sleeping bag up and put it in its waterproof case, put his boots on, then crawled out of his tent. Of course, it was damp, but he pulled up the stakes and shook it sharply. With as much of the rain off it as possible, he folded it and pushed it into the carrying bag along with the stakes. When he arrived at his house was soon enough to spread it out to get it dry.

He barely had his gear ready for the trail when the cook called, "Breakfast's ready, come now before it gets cold and soggy!"

"Bless her!" he said fervently.

"We're after it, Tillie!" someone yelled.

Everyone hurried, nearly gulping down their food. By seven o'clock everyone had their rain slickers on, their backpacks in place and they were moving down the slippery trail. As during the other hurricane, they moved as fast as the conditions permitted, keeping as close together as the trail allowed. All morning, each of them snacked on granola bars and trail mix as they became hungry, because Ramon had told them they wouldn't be stopping for a regular lunch break, only momentarily at a stream to purify water for their canteens. Nobody complained they wanted to get home as soon as possible.

Ramon was in the lead with Duncan taking up the last place and everyone else straggled along in between. Ramon had his eyes on the clouds as often as he could, while he watched the trail because he wasn't familiar with it, except to look at it before they'd left on Duncan's computer screen. It wasn't too rugged and as he remembered, there wasn't any shale, but the trail wandered through the forest.

Since the rain started during the night, there had been no break in the rain, sometimes it rained harder than other times and some of those times it rained very hard. Ramon looked at his watch, thinking about Sandy at the office. It was eleven thirty and he glanced up at the clouds again. They were ominous, churning and turning green. Ramon's ears strained to listen, but what he heard sent a shiver down his back.

"Everybody hit the ground, roll for the nearest depression! A tornado's about to hit us! Down, everyone!" he yelled against the wind.

Ramon turned around and dropped to his knees, wanting to make sure all those in the group heard him and were doing as he said. Duncan was last and he'd seen the green, turbulent clouds, so he yelled to those in front of him, "Down! Hit the ground!"

Just as Ramon threw himself onto the ground the roar went over, but with it went one of the tall trees. The roots only skimmed along the ground, but began to climb as the tornado sucked it up. The root system was dragging great clods of dirt along with stones. One of the larger clods contained a large rock and it dropped from the root system just as it passed over Ramon. The rock fell squarely on Ramon's head. His vision became fuzzy immediately, but he fought to keep his mind clear.

Almost as soon as the roar came, it left, but Ramon was down, his head was swimming and he had a massive headache. He felt the gray clouding his vision and he felt himself loosing consciousness, things moved in slow motion and sounds seemed far away, but Duncan scrambled up and rolled him onto his back.

"Tell me what to do!" he yelled, frantic.

"Cell phone...push one...tell Sandy... to call Fisher........she'll know..."

The black hole swallowed Ramon.

With shaking hands, Duncan pushed up Ramon's slicker and grabbed the phone from his belt. The youth pastor pulled the slicker down, covering Ramon as much as possible. The tornado was long gone, but the rain poured down, the wind was fierce. Duncan's hands trembled so much he nearly dropped the slippery little phone before he had it so he could see the face and the buttons. His hands trembling, he punched the one key and held the phone to his ear. When nothing happened, he pulled it away and punched the one again. Finally, after the third time he thought to push the ON button and then punch the one. He never thought to look at his watch.

Sandy looked at the clock on the desk and gathered her things to put in the drawer, it was five to twelve, but nearly as dark as night. She looked out at the rain and the ominous clouds, wishing she was home already. She wanted to get started on Ramon's favorite meal she'd have spaghetti with meatballs and garlic bread.

The phone rang, and her heart tripped over itself, the last time in a rain like this, it was Ramon and someone on his hike was hurt. "Hello?"

"Sandy!" a frantic voice yelled, "Duncan! Ramon said to call Fisher!"

"Someone's hurt?"

"Yes, Ramon! Hurry, he's unconscious now!"

Trying to keep her own panic at bay, Sandy said, "Duncan, listen to me!" It was obvious that the man was frantic and perhaps not thinking clearly. "Duncan, disconnect, but don't turn off the phone. Fisher will call you in a minute to get your location. When you've given it, disconnect, leave someone with Ramon, then you lead the rest of the group out. I'll call you back in fifteen minutes."

"Yes!"

Sandy pushed the disconnect button and dropped the phone on the desk. Her heart was beating so fast and hard it felt like it would fly out of her chest. Her hands were trembling, but in that instant her only thought was to pray. "Father in heaven! Please be with Ramon, I don't know what happened but be with him, put Your hands of love and protection around him. And Father, help me to do the right thing. Please let Fisher be there and help me tell him the right thing." As she prayed out loud, Sandy's hands found the phone book, opened it to the back cover and ran her finger down the page. Fisher's name was in bold letters and the numbers were bold. Her hands trembling, she picked up the phone again and dialed the number in front of her.

"MEDIVAC," the voice answered immediately.

"I just got a frantic call from Ramon DeLord's group. There's been some injury. They are expecting your call to give location." She gave the man Ramon's cellphone number and hung up. The tears she'd felt ever since she'd heard Duncan's frantic voice slid down her face.

"God, my Father, be with him!"

Duncan couldn't pace with all the hikers around him, but he wanted to. He looked at the phone in his hand several times, but thought it would never ring. It did, only a few minutes later, but it seemed like hours. "Hello!"

The calm voice on the other end, said, "This is MEDIVAC. I understand you have an injury that needs airlifting."

"Yes, our leader, Ramon DeLord was hit with debris following a tornado, he's unconscious and we can't seem to rouse him!"

"Can you give me your location?"

Duncan was hunched over the papers he'd printed from his computer, trying to read them in the rain and wind and finally was able to see one of the landmarks. His hands were trembling so much the papers were rattling, but he told the man the landmark he saw. The rescuer said, "Okay, we've located you on our map and someone is suiting up now, he'll be there in a few minutes. Can someone act as the leader without Ramon?"

Duncan took a deep breath, knowing that responsibility now rested on him. After another deep breath, he said, "Yes, I'm Duncan Roads; I'm going to start working with Ramon on a regular basis, so I will be. I'm new around here, should I wait with Ramon until you folks arrive or head the group out?"

"Here's what we've done in the past. Designate someone to stay with Ramon and you continue your hike back to headquarters. We'll take Ramon and whoever stays with him and their gear. The chopper is ready and the pilot's on the run."

"Thank you!" Duncan said his relief was palpable in the words. Duncan disconnected, looked around for the leader and said, "Mr. Ways, do you have someone who can stay with Ramon while the rest of us hike out?"

The pastor found his oldest young man and said, "David, come stay with Ramon. Someone will be coming to lift him and you out. The rest of us will go with Duncan."

All the young people were milling around the tiny clearing. They were scared now that the tornado had come through and especially since Ramon had been hurt, but Duncan said, "Get your packs on guys, we're moving on. We need to get back to base as soon as possible. The helicopter will be here soon for Ramon."

They had barely moved when the phone rang again. Duncan answered and Sandy said, "Did they call you?"

"Yes, someone was leaving as we spoke. Sandy thanks for being so level-headed. You helped me focus on what I needed to do. We're on our way now." Even before he finished speaking they heard the familiar sound of the helicopter blades. He said into the phone, "That was fast! The chopper just went over."

"Good! Duncan, do you need to get back in the office when you get here?"

"I can't think of a reason except to leave the phone."

"That's fine, I want to go to the hospital, so put the phone in the mailbox next to the office door. I'll get it tomorrow."

"I'll do that, Sandy. Thanks."

Sandy hung up, flipped the phone to the answering machine, grabbed her rain slicker and threw it over her head. As it slithered down her back, she pulled the plastic over her lap. She killed the lights and locked the door, then pushed the control button to the fastest forward position on her chair. In her other hand she had the key for her van door ready to open it. Neither the door nor the lift moved very fast, but finally, she was inside. All the plastic was cumbersome so she shed the plastic lap cover and the slicker on the back seat then locked her chair behind the steering wheel. She sighed, if the chopper had gone over while she'd been talking to Duncan, Ramon was probably already at the hospital. She was very glad this system for emergencies had already been set up. They could be caring for Ramon already.

There were two men in the chopper, the pilot and a paramedic. They saw the localized devastation of the tornado and were surprised that Ramon had been the only one who'd been hit. Ramon and the young man from the youth group were easy to see, their rain slickers were both bright yellow. The chopper slowed and carefully settled. The rain didn't let up it was torrential as the pilot slacked off on the engine.

The rotors were still beating the air, but the paramedic was on the ground. Ramon hadn't moved since Duncan had rolled him on his back. The pastor had positioned his backpack so that the rain wouldn't hit him squarely in the face, but the young man was pacing a few feet back and forth, each time he came close to Ramon, he looked down at him, but he hadn't touched him.

The paramedic said, "What happened?"

"A tornado went through. He yelled for us to lie down and roll, but he stayed on his knees until he was sure we were all down." The young man pointed to the rock close by. "When a tree was sucked up in the tornado, the roots pulled up dirt and all. That rock fell as it went over Ramon and got him real good."

"Nothing else?"

David shook his head. "No, not that I know of."

The paramedic put a neck brace around Ramon's neck and told the young man, "Take your two packs to the chopper and climb in. My friend and I'll get Ramon inside."

The young man gratefully nodded. "Thanks," he said.

He did as he was told and moved the packs to a place that obviously was meant for cargo. David stayed with them until the other two men had Ramon inside and onto the fastened down stretcher. Even with all the movement, Ramon didn't move any part of his body, groan or make any sound. Both the pilot and the paramedic were surprised, they'd expected that all the movement would wake him or cause him to groan.

As the three men strapped in, the pilot asked, "Did anyone notify Ramon's mom? Was she the one who called in?"

"No, before he went out cold Ramon told Duncan to call Sandy."

"Sandy?"

"Yeah, his receptionist. I guess she called you."

"Hmm, would she have called his mom?"

"I don't know."

The pilot pushed the stick so that the chopper rose sharply, then he turned to his sidekick and said, "Maybe you'd better give the woman a call. She should be the one to give info and permission if it's needed. Activate the directory on the phone. I think her name's Casbah now."

"I'm scrolling down now."

They were in the air when Millie answered and a voice said, "Mrs. Casbah? This is MEDIVAC. We're airlifting your son to Blairsville Hospital. He's been injured on the trail."

"No! Oh, no! You're sure it's Ramon?"

"Ma'am, I'm a friend of Ramon's I know the man when I see him."

"Blairsville Hospital? I'll be there!"

"Thank you, Ma'am," the young man said over the drone of the chopper. However, he said it to a dial tone.

Sandy recognized Millie's Jag as she skidded around a corner in front of her. Sandy sighed, she should have thought to call Millie, but obviously MEDIVAC had done it. Millie pulled her car up under the covering at the front door. Sandy saw her and knew she shouldn't park there. Sandy went to the parking garage and parked in a handicapped spot, let her lift down and quickly wheeled herself out, locked up and hurried to the elevator to take to the floor where the bridge was.

Inside, she wheeled herself up to the information desk and said to the woman, "Where would they bring a person airlifted here by MEDIVAC?"

"Back to the emergency department, Ma'am! Follow the blue line on the wall, it'll lead you right there."

Sandy set her chair in motion and said over her shoulder, "Thanks."

The lady smiled and said, "Not a problem!"

The pilot set his chopper down only inches from the covered receiving area. He had radioed in, so hospital personnel were waiting. The paramedic helped the hospital people to take Ramon out then David dragged the two heavy backpacks out with him. The paramedic motioned for him to come in the elevator with them as they took Ramon down to the main floor. The elevator was a non-stop directly to the ER. Usually when the helicopter was sent out it was for an emergency. Everything was geared for it.

Millie came crashing into the waiting room as the elevator doors opened. Instead of going to the information desk, she ran to the stretcher where Ramon was strapped down. As she looked down at him, tears streamed down her cheeks. She grabbed his limp hand and cried, "Ramon, my son!" She looked up at the man pulling the head of the stretcher. "What's the matter with him?"

"A rock knocked him out."

"A rock?"

"Yes, his hiking group was in a tornado and a flying rock hit him."

"Oh, my!"

"Ma'am, please go to the desk, you'll need to give some information about him."

Millie looked down again at her son, chewed on her bottom lip, then finally turned from the stretcher and headed back to the desk. She was giving information as Sandy wheeled herself into the department and saw the stretcher before they had it in an exam room. She wheeled herself over, but stayed out of the way. Of course, those at MEDIVAC had heard her voice twice, but had never seen her. The two men wheeling Ramon's stretcher both scowled at her, but didn't comment.

When they had him in the room and came out, Sandy said, "Excuse me, has he woken from being unconscious yet?"

The paramedic said nothing, but the hospital man said, "You a relative?"

"No, I work for Ramon."

The man shook his head. "Can't tell you anything, only family."

The paramedic finally said, "Ma'am, that kid over there with the backpacks was there, you might ask him."

Sandy smiled at him and said, "Thanks, I'll do that." Even though Sandy wanted to be with Ramon, she set her chair on a course to find out what happened. She smiled at the young man and asked, "What happened?"

"A tornado went over. A tree was uprooted and the roots held a huge rock until it was right over Ramon's head, then the rock let loose and fell right on his head. He stayed awake long enough to tell Duncan what to do, then he lost consciousness."

"Wow!" Sandy said.

Millie was distracted and barely answered questions before she rushed over as a doctor started to enter Ramon's room. She brushed by him, forcing him to wait for her to enter first. She never glanced at him, but rushed up and grabbed Ramon's hand. A nurse was already in the room pulling off Ramon's slicker and unbuttoning his shirt. She didn't look at Millie.

"What are you doing to my son?" Millie demanded of the woman.

"Ma'am, we always make sure there's no constricting clothing on a patient. The doctor will want to check his lungs and also make a total inspection. If you'll step back into the waiting room, we can complete our examination more quickly."

"I won't leave my son!" Millie screamed at the woman and sent an elbow into her ribs. "You can't make me leave him!"

The younger woman stopped what she was doing and turned around. She took Millie's arm and kindly, but forcibly took her from the room. "Yes, Ma'am, you will. We need to be able to move around the room easily. At this point we have no idea how extensive his injuries are and we don't need you fainting on us, too."

"I thought you needed my permission to work on him!" she said, petulantly.

"Ma'am, you signed that release when you gave us the information at the desk."

"Oh." Millie saw Sandy, but didn't go to her she sank into the nearest chair.

Sandy talked with the young man from the youth group who was getting more and more agitated. He was hoping his group would come by for him, but Sandy assured him that it was a much slower process to walk the trails back to Ramon's office than to be airlifted to the hospital.

When she saw the nurse bring Millie from the room, she said to the young man, "Come on, bring those packs and let's go over to those chairs. That's Ramon's mom sitting over there, surely we can come up with something to talk about together." Sandy wheeled herself up beside Millie and David followed her, still pulling the heavy backpacks behind him.

David left the wet packs on the floor on the other side of Millie then flopped into the next chair, with a long sigh. Millie didn't acknowledge either Sandy or David, but the leg she had crossed over her other knee was waving back and forth furiously. This was the first time Sandy had seen Millie in less than pristine condition.

Moments later, the doctor came over and asked, "Are you three here with Ramon?"

Millie jumped up, exclaiming, "Yes, oh, yes! What do you know? What could have happened to my son?"

Looking at the nearly hysterical woman, he said, "He has a severe concussion that caused him to loose consciousness. Since he hasn't come to, I'll admit him. Are you his mother?"

"Yes! Yes, of course! If you need him to stay with someone when he wakes up, I have a big house, I'll be glad to take him home."

The doctor smiled at her. "We'll work on that after he wakes up, but thanks." He looked at the other two people. "Any relative?"

"No, I work for Ramon and this young man was there when Ramon was hit and stayed with him and came in the helicopter with him."

The man shook his head and said apologetically, "I'm sorry, then, I can't let but his mother in to see him right now."

Sandy smiled, but swallowed and said, "I guess we'll live with that."

The nurse hurried from the room before the doctor left, looked at him, then at the other three and said, "Is anyone of you Sandy?"

Sandy smiled, "Yes, I'm Sandy."

The nurse smiled at Sandy and said, "The patient is asking for Sandy. He hasn't regained consciousness, but he's asking for Sandy." The nurse raised her hand as if to motion to Sandy, then thought to say, "Doctor, should I let her in?"

"Of course! If the young man's asking for her then let her in. He'll probably respond to her voice more quickly than any other."

Sandy looked gratefully at the doctor and pushed her control forward to take her into the room. Millie still sat in the chair and whined, "How about me? Can I go in?"

The nurse said, "Ma'am lets see if he will respond and wake up to Sandy's voice. If he does, I'll come for you."

"I should go in!" she muttered. "I'm his mother. His mother should be the one to be with him when he's hurt!"

"Ma'am," the nurse said sternly, "he's asked for Sandy."

Sandy wasn't concerned about Millie, since Ramon was calling for her and she could hear him. She wheeled up beside him and took his hand. She bent over, but the bed he lay on was so high that she couldn't reach his face at all. The nurse turned and saw the dilemma, so she came immediately and lowered the bed several inches.

Sandy smiled at her then mouthed the words, "Thank you!" As soon as the bed was low enough, she bent over again and kissed him on the lips. "Ramon, I heard you calling for me. Wake up! You're here at the hospital and we all want you to wake up. You're being lazy, you know." Her last sentence she said with a smile in her voice, she'd heard that an unconscious person responded better to cheerfulness than sorrowfulness. "Come on, now, don't be lazy!"

He was in a black place, it felt like the middle of a tunnel and there were invisible strings holding him inside. He called, hoping someone would hear him and come to help him get free. "Sandy! Sandy!" *It was still black, but maybe one of the strings tying his leg had broken, something had changed.* "Sandy! Sandy!"

"I'm here, Ramon, come on, wake up! You've had a long enough nap, it's time you woke up and quit lying around."

Ramon didn't open his eyes, but turned his head toward her voice and groaned, "Sandy?"

"Yes, I'm here." She bent over and kissed his lips again.

"Mmm, do that again," he murmured, still with his eyes closed.

"Can you open your eyes for me?"

She watched and his eyes moved behind his eyelids, but they didn't open. "Okay, if you can't open your eyes, can you squeeze my hand?"

Ramon's fingers moved, but he didn't apply any pressure to her hand. Sandy looked up at the nurse, who was scowling. "What you're asking isn't computing."

Sandy nodded. "Yes, that seems to be it."

The nurse pushed a button on the wall and when a voice answered, she said, "Call Dr. Ambrose and tell him we need a consult in room G."

"He's here at the desk, he'll be right there."

Soon the man entered. "Yes, what is it?"

The nurse continued to look at Ramon, but she said, "He's called for Sandy several times and she answered as soon as she was in the room, he acknowledged her once. She kissed him, he asked for a repeat. She asked him to open his eyes, his eyes moved under his lids, but they didn't open. When she asked him to squeeze her hand, his fingers moved but he didn't make any attempt to squeeze her hand."

"Hmm, that's interesting." The man turned to Sandy and said, "Call him by name and tell him who you are."

"Ramon, this is Sandy, it's time to wake up." All three in the room watched, but nothing happened. Ramon didn't groan or move.

The doctor shook his head. "He must have lapsed back."

Fearfully, Sandy asked, "Is that normal?"

"It happens as often as not. Lets admit him. I've called up to the medical ward they have a bed for him. Miss...I don't know your name?"

"I'm Sandy Bernard. We work quite closely together."

"Sandy Bernard! I thought you looked familiar!" the doctor exclaimed. "You played that lovely concert in Vansville the other night."

"Yes, I did."

"And this is Ramon, the MC."

"Yes, you're right again."

The man held out his hand and smiled. "Believe me, I was impressed. Okay. We'll send him upstairs and keep close watch on him. Since he called for you, can you stay with him?"

"Of course!"

Millie heard the people talking in Ramon's room, so she rushed to the door and looked in. "Did you wake him up yet?"

"No, Ma'am, he seemed to respond for a few minutes, but now he doesn't. We're having him transferred upstairs."

"I'm his mother, wouldn't he respond to me?"

"Possibly, but if an unconscious person calls for someone by name we usually ask that person to try to rouse him. He hasn't asked for his mom, not one time."

She stamped her high heeled shoe and whined, "That's not fair! She shouldn't be able to be with him! After all, she's no relation to him."

"I'm sorry, Ma'am, she was who he called for. I'm sure you can try after we get him settled in a room upstairs.

Millie glared at Sandy, who smiled back, but neither the nurse nor the doctor noticed the exchange, they were busy getting Ramon ready for being moved. Only moments later, a young man came to the door with a stretcher and said to Millie, "Excuse me I need to wheel this in so we can get the patient on here."

Millie glared at the young man, but finally stepped one step outside the room, but she said, "Okay, but make her move, too. She'll surely be in the way with that chair and all." The woman's sarcasm was totally lost on the man with the stretcher.

Sandy had moved to the head of the emergency room bed, so when the young man looked up, he said, "She's not in the way at all."

Frustrated, Millie kicked the door frame, which was steel and she yelled, "Owe!" However, no one paid any attention to her.

By this time, David, the young man who'd come with Ramon was pacing in the waiting room. He felt lost, very much out of his comfort zone. He kept an eye on the two backpacks, but he was anxious for his friends and pastor to come for him. He looked around as Millie yelled, but he mostly watched the door coming in from outside.

When everyone came from the room, following Ramon on the stretcher, Sandy asked the nurse, "That young man came with Ramon on the MEDIVAC helicopter. He's with a group of hikers and they'll have to come for him. What should he do until then?"

"Let me talk to him. You'd better take Ramon's backpack upstairs."

"Sure, I'll get it."

The small elevator, headed for the medical floor was quite crowded, the young man with Ramon's stretcher went on first,

Sandy grabbed Ramon's backpack and brought it on with her onto the elevator and Millie, of course would not be left behind. Millie wouldn't speak to Sandy, but whenever she looked at her she glared at her.

In the elevator, Ramon groaned, threw an arm over his eyes and said, "Sandy! Sandy!"

She couldn't get to his head, but she touched his hand and said, "I'm here, Ramon. We're moving you to a bed in the hospital."

"Hospital?"

"Yes, we're leaving the Emergency Room we're in the elevator going to a room so you can stay overnight."

"Why?"

"Because you've been napping for over two hours and you have a huge goose egg on your head. The doctor says you have a concussion from the rock that hit you."

Ramon groaned. "I remember now. A tornado."

Moving just as close as she could in the cramped space, she said, "Yes, it took out a tree close by and a rock fell from the roots and dropped on you. The doctor wants to make sure you'll be okay before he sends you home."

Ramon's eyelids felt like lead. He wanted to see where he was and what was going on, but his lids wouldn't open, even though he willed them to several times. As he lay visualizing where he was his thoughts turned to Sandy. She'd come through for him again. She'd followed directions both times there'd been trouble. He'd been convinced before, but he knew it deep in his soul, he loved this woman, she was his better half. They were moving he could feel the movement. He could hear the soft whine of Sandy's chair and she was holding his hand. Someone else was going with them, another female hand held his other one. That woman hadn't said anything, but he guessed it was his mom. He could hear the click of her heels.

"Ramon, we must let go of your hands, the man needs to push you through the door. As soon as you're in the bed we'll be back."

"Mom?"

"Yes, Darling, I'm right here!" Millie said, dramatically.

"Mom, go on home!"

"No! No, I won't be leaving until you do!"

"I don't think so! It's enough to have Sandy here." The woman stamped her foot, but didn't say anything. The look on her face was enough of a response. Again, it was lost on Ramon, since his eyes were closed.

The young man wheeled the stretcher through the doorway onto the ward then down the hallway to the room and up beside the bed. There was a nurse already in the room, so the two hospital personnel moved Ramon onto the bed. The nurse covered him, while the man took the stretcher back through the door and disappeared down the hall toward the elevator.

The nurse said to Ramon, "So, can you open your eyes for me?"

Ramon tried to will his eyelids to open and finally there was a tiny sliver of light as they moved a little. He groaned, "The light's really bright. Do I have to open them more?"

"Is that your girlfriend out in the hall?"

"Sandy's there. I want her."

Sandy sat beside the door, close enough to hear Ramon's exchange with the nurse, but Millie blocked the doorway once the man with the stretcher left. It was a warrior stance, she had her arms crossed over her chest, but her elbows spread and her legs, even in her high heels were stretched apart. "Is he settled? Can I go in?" she demanded. "It's my right!"

"Are you Sandy?"

"No! I'm his mom. I demand to be allowed in with him! This is the most ridiculous thing I've ever heard of!"

"I'm sorry, Ma'am, he asked for Sandy. Visitors aren't restricted on this floor. I suppose you can go in as well."

SIXTEEN

Millie stepped around the young woman immediately and pushed on the door to close it. The nurse scowled, but then pushed the door back open and said to Sandy, "He asked for you, so you'd better get in there."

"Thank you."

Sandy wheeled in, but Ramon was already speaking to his mom, so she sat back out of the way. "Mom! I realize you had to give information and permission since I was unconscious when I first came in. However, now that you've done that you can go. I want to spend this time with Sandy. It surely has to be supper time, go home and eat your dinner with Derek."

"I will not leave you!"

"You had better not get me riled, Mom. I have a mind to call security on you."

"You wouldn't dare!"

"Yes, I would, Mom. I want Sandy right here, right beside me." He took a breath and asked, "Sandy, are you here?"

"Yes, Ramon, I'm here."

"Please, come up here beside me on this other side."

Millie was angry and humiliated when Ramon turned his back on her and turned, even with his eyes closed toward Sandy. "Sandy, Love, thanks for everything." He wished he could pull her up onto the bed with him.

He held out his hand to her and she grasped it, but she said, "Ramon, I did nothing out of the ordinary! Duncan called and I called MEDIVAC, then I came here!"

Millie huffed, as she heard the endearment Ramon used. She had been standing beside the bed, but when she heard what he called her, she threw herself onto the foot of the bed, bouncing up and down a few times intentionally. Whether she knew it or not, she jounced Ramon's head, drawing out a groan from him. Millie hated being ignored and Ramon and Sandy were certainly ignoring her.

"Mom, I want to be alone with Sandy. Please leave," he commanded.

"As long as she's here, so am I!"

"No, Mom, that's not the way it works. I'm a grown man now. I make up my own mind as to who I want to be with. Now that I'm conscious and know what's going on, I want to be alone with Sandy. She'll be here for quite a while, but you are leaving now. If you don't, I have the call button right here and I'll tell the desk to send security."

"Well!" She deliberately bounced on the bed several times before sliding off. The movement made Ramon's head throb and he groaned. She ignored it, however, and said, "I can tell when I'm not wanted. You won't let me come to your house any more, now you don't want me here, even though you were hurt so badly. You'll hire a nurse to come stay with you when the doctor releases you? I offered to take you home."

"I'll see to it, Mom! Don't trouble yourself."

Finally, the troublesome woman left. They could hear her heels clicking on the tiled hallway floor. With the dim light over his bed and only Sandy in the room who knew how to keep quiet if it was necessary, he tried to open his eyes again. This time, they came open almost all the way. He was on his side and she filled his vision. His smile was only the raising of one side of his mouth, but Sandy's heart tripped over itself as she saw it.

"You still feel bad, don't you?" she asked.

"Lets say I've felt better. One hundred percent better would almost bring it up to normal." He squeezed her hand and said, "Didn't you kiss me down in the ER?"

She blushed. "Yes, but you didn't wake up."

"No, I fell back into the black hole, but I remember that I did ask you to do that again. Will you now?"

"Of course!" He held her hand, but she wheeled her chair close and covered his mouth.

That was how the house doctor found them. "I see she's done her job, she woke you up."

"Yeah, that she has!" Ramon said, a bit breathlessly.

The phone rang beside the bed, but Ramon was turned toward Sandy who sat on the opposite side of the bed from the phone. The doctor reached for the receiver and said, "Hello?"

"Umm, this is Duncan Roads. I was told that Ramon DeLord was in this room."

"You have the right place. I'm his doctor, but he's tied up with a lady right now."

"So he's woken up?"

On a chuckle, the doctor said, "Yes, this same young lady kissed him awake, I do believe. He's a bit incapacitated right now, though."

"That's okay. Will you tell him and her, that we got back to his office about half an hour ago. The group left to pick up their friend there at Blairsville Hospital. I left the phone where Sandy said to leave it and we've all left his place."

"I'll spread the word," the doctor said. "They'll be glad to know things are all set."

"Thanks."

The doctor hung up and relayed the message, then he said, "So, your mom will take you home when I release you?"

Shaking his head, then realized that was a bad idea and stopped immediately, Ramon said, "Not that I'm aware, Doc. She asked if I'd hire a nurse to stay with me when you discharge me. That sounds like a better idea, believe me."

The doctor scowled, looking from the young man to the lady in the wheelchair. "She told me she has a big house and she'll take you home."

"I guess she said that when I was still out, because I didn't hear that. No, after I kicked her out of here, on her way through the door, she asked if I'd hire a nurse. If that's what needs to be done, that's what'll happen."

"You don't get along?"

Ramon's head moved a little, but stopped, as he said, "We haven't in a long time, Doc. You're keeping me here over night. I have my own house and Sandy'll be there in the morning. She can take me home from here tomorrow."

Dr. Ambrose scowled, and asked Sandy, "You drive?"

"Yes, I do. When will you release him?"

The man rubbed his chin and said, "Probably after breakfast. I'll come by and make sure everything's okay before I write the order."

Sandy nodded. "I'll be here."

"That'll be fine."

After the doctor left, Sandy said, "Ramon, you know you antagonized your mom again. She'll never know about your new relationship with Christ that way."

Ramon took both of her hands, then looked deeply into her eyes and said, "Sweetheart, we haven't really liked each other for a long time. I think she blamed me, not herself, for my dad leaving us. Paint your picture for her and you show her Christ. I'll back you up, but I really doubt she'll listen to me. She'll try to smother me, but she won't listen."

The nurse stuck her head in the door and asked, "Mr. DeLord, could you eat?"

"Could I eat! I haven't had a good meal since last night's supper! I think I could eat a brimming pot of Sandy's spaghetti and not feel too full."

"How about you, Ma'am?"

"Yes, if it's not too much trouble."

"The doctor ordered you supper, so I'll call down orders for two meals."

"Thanks, that won't make us mad," Ramon assured the woman.

"Great! Your trays'll be up in a few minutes."

In the morning, Sandy hurried with her routine and arrived at the hospital about eight. She parked in the covered place in front of the main entrance. A man in a blue uniform came around her van, but Sandy didn't see him and was opening the door to let herself down on the lift when he reached the driver's door. He scowled, taken aback by the fact there was no one in the driver's seat, but also there was no seat. Then he wondered where she had disappeared to. Finally, he heard the noise of her lift extending.

He came back around as Sandy was lowering herself to the pavement. He was still scowling as he said, "Are you seeing a doctor, Ma'am?"

Of course, Sandy smiled at the man. "No, Sir, I'm picking up a man who's being discharged. It'll only be here a few minutes."

"All right, fine. This time of morning there's not too much activity through here, but don't dilly dally!"

"Thank you, sir."

Only a few minutes later Sandy wheeled herself beside the wheelchair the CNA used to bring Ramon out the front door. The woman looked at Sandy's van and said, "This is cool! You can drive yourself, can't you?"

Smiling, because someone had really understood her, Sandy said, "Yes, I'm really glad I can. It makes me feel a little independent."

"I can believe that."

Finally, they were in the van, Ramon in the passenger seat and of course, Sandy was behind the wheel. "How do you feel this morning?"

"Like I've been run over by a Mac Truck."

"I'll stay with you all day."

Ramon sighed. "I'm so glad, Sandy. I really didn't want to be alone, but I'm not about to call Mom to come."

When Sandy had the van on the highway going back to Vansville, Ramon said, "Sweetheart, I love you. Do you think you could ever love me?"

The pull off where Sandy had painted Ramon's picture was just ahead and Sandy wheeled into it. She stopped the van, put it in park, unlocked her chair and brought herself as close to him as she could come. "Say that again?" she asked, incredulous.

He swiveled on the seat, took her hands and held them, then brought them to his lips and kissed each finger. He looked into her eyes, hoping she could see all the love he had for her reflected there. "I love you, Sweetheart. Do you think you could ever love me?"

She looked at their hands their fingers entwined, then looked into his eyes. Earnestly, she said, "You love me? Ramon, I'm crippled I sit in a wheelchair for sixteen or more hours every day. I always have, I always will. You love me? Like this?" She shook her head. "I never thought I was someone anybody could love."

"I wouldn't lie to you! I love you the way you are. You aren't crippled! You were paralyzed as a baby, so you sit in a wheelchair, but Darling, you're more alive than most people who have four extremities that work. Of course I love you!"

"You love me? You love *me*! YOU LOVE ME! I can't believe it! Could I ever love you? Could I! Ramon, oh, yes, yes! I love you with all my heart!"

His hands slid up her arms, gently pulling her toward him. She leaned as far toward him as she could and he closed the gap. Their arms circled each other and his lips claimed hers. It was a special kiss, one sealing their love for each other. This time when his tongue touched her lower lip and she gasped, he brought his tongue against her teeth and her mouth opened to him. He lazily ran his tongue past her teeth and touched her tongue. She gasped again, and pulled back, her hands leaving the back of his neck, but grasping tightly to his shoulders.

"Why did you do that?" she gasped out the words.

"Because I love you. Darling, would you marry me?"

Incredulous, she looked at him, moisture collecting in her eyes and a warm rush covered her whole body. "You... You're throwing things at me so fast! Ramon, I've never done that before... I mean, had a kiss like that before. Umm, you want to marry me? This is all so incredible! I never thought anyone would look at me much because of this chair. I can't believe you can love me, but you want to marry me, too?"

"Sandy!" Ramon almost came out of the seat, but his headache was so bad, he fell back in the bucket seat. "Sandy! Believe me! I want to spend the rest of my life loving you and making you happy!"

"But I am happy!" She looked deep into his eyes, her eyes clear a window to her soul. "You really want to marry me?"

Ramon nodded. "That's the desire of my heart, Sweetheart. I want to spend every day for the rest of my life with you – loving you."

"Ramon, if you're sure, my answer is yes!"

Ramon did come out of the seat then. He put his hand on the control of her chair and moved it so they could go to the back of the van. When they reached the back bench, he slid his hands around her, one around her shoulders and one under her legs and lifted her from the chair. He whirled around and sat down with Sandy on his lap then he began to kiss her properly. Many minutes passed while they were on the back seat. Ramon felt he'd never been happier in all his life, as he was at that moment. He completely forgot about his pounding head.

When Sandy turned onto Ramon's driveway, the Jag already sat on the parking lot. Millie obviously had already knocked on the office door she was standing at the front door knocking on it. Ramon let out a long frustrated breath as he saw her. He wanted Sandy not even to stop, but to turn around and head for her cabin.

Millie, of course, heard the van and immediately abandoned the front door. She ran as best she could in her tight skirt and spike heels, to the front door of the van. "Ramon! You let her bring you home? Why didn't you call me?"

Trying to hold in his frustration, he said, "Because I wanted Sandy to bring me home. Besides, we had some important words to say to each other."

"What *could* that be?"

With a grin, Ramon answered without hesitation, "Sandy has agreed to be my wife! This is the happiest day of my life!"

Rain was still pelting down Millie's hair was getting plastered to her head, her mascara running rivers down her face. "What? What! WHAT!! You're going to marry *her*?"

"Yes, Mom, I surely am! We've decided that as soon as we can get everyone to agree on a date that we'll get married and Sandy will move here."

"You don't mean this!" Tears welled up in her eyes and slid down through her eye makeup. "You *can't* mean that!"

Still with a grin wider than the Mississippi, and holding Sandy's hand up so Millie could see him holding it, he said, "Yes, Mom, I've never been more serious in my life. I love Sandy and she loves me. We want to share our lives from now on."

"Oh, my! Oh, my!" Millie swiped at her eyes, smearing the mascara on her cheek, but the tears kept running down. Her perfect son was ruining her plans. How could he do such a thing to her? He couldn't, just couldn't!

Oblivious to Millie's thoughts, Ramon continued, "The doctor informed me today that I can't lead a hike until he's satisfied that everything's okay. He said that'll be at least a week, that's when I'm to see him again. I'm going to call Duncan and see if he wants to start early as my associate and lead the rest of the groups this season. We'll also call Sandy's parents. We're hoping they'll say yes, but we're planning on taking our honeymoon along the way to Philadelphia. It'll be our gift to each other."

Millie looked at Sandy, accusation in her voice, "You said you'd marry my son?"

"Yes, I have," Sandy said. "I love him very much, Mrs. Casbah."

Millie shook her head and turned from the van. They both heard her say, "I never imagined something like this would ever happen." Fortunately, she kept most of the words she wanted to say from coming out. Without another word, Millie turned and walked to her Jag. The rain pouring down had soaked her completely. All her clothes were plastered to her. She never looked back, just opened the door, slid in and started up. In minutes she was gone.

Sandy went to her lift and pushed the inside controls. Ramon was slow to move from the seat, he wanted to be sure his mom was gone from the parking lot before he stepped out. He heard the powerful engine roar into life and heard the tires squeal as she made tracks off the parking lot. Again this time she made a wider swing than needed and almost hit Sandy's van.

Ramon sighed, as Sandy came to the door, "I hope she's gone for good! If she expected me to call her to come for me at the hospital, why'd she come here? If she expected me to hire a nurse to come here when I was released, why'd she come here?"

Sandy chuckled. "I have no answer to either of your questions. Does a mother always think rationally about her child?"

"When you say it that way, I don't think so."

Sandy saw how pale he was, so she said, "If you need to hold onto my chair, be sure you do. I'll go as slowly as you need to."

"Thanks, Sweetheart," he sighed. "I've felt lots better in my life."

"I know, I can tell easily, Honey."

That evening after a delicious meal Sandy fixed at Ramon's house and he had eaten a generous portion even for seconds, Ramon picked up the cordless phone from the office and brought it in to the kitchen where Sandy was finishing supper clean-up. Sandy draped the dish cloth over the sink, lifted the phone from the wall receptacle and came back to the table, to sit close to Ramon. He held the cordless in his hand, but Sandy dialed a long distance number. While it rang, Ramon turned his on.

"Hello, Bernards."

"Hi, Mom, is Daddy so he can get an extension?"

They heard another click and the voice said, "Sandy?"

"Hi, Daddy. I have some really great news I want to share with you both. Mom and Dad, Ramon has asked me to marry him...."

Colleen gasped and before she covered the mouthpiece they both heard a strangled, "No-o-o-o! No! NO!"

Undaunted, Sandy said, "Yes, Mom, he asked me yesterday and I've told him, 'yes' that I would. Daddy, Mom, I love Ramon and he loves me..."

"I'm..." Charlie started.

"But you can't!" Colleen cried.

"Why?"

"You just can't! You mustn't! I knew something terrible was happening down there! You must come home immediately!"

Speaking to her mom as one grown woman to another, Sandy said, "No, Mom, I'm a grown woman. I can get married nothing terrible is happening down here. I won't be coming to Philadelphia immediately, not until after our wedding and then only for our honeymoon."

"No, no, NO!"

Both Sandy and Ramon heard something through the receiver and Charlie spoke, "Sandy, is your Ramon there?"

"Yes, Daddy, he's here listening on another phone."

The older man could hear the tears in his daughter's voice. He hated that her mom had put a damper on their daughter's happiness. He swallowed and said, "Sandy, I took the phone from your mama. We'll work this out after we hang up. When will you have the ceremony?"

"Very soon, Daddy, we don't see any reason to wait. Ramon was hurt yesterday, so he can't lead any hikes for at least a week until he sees the doctor again. The doctor didn't sound positive even then. We're trying to reach his associate to see if he will take over, then we'll decide for sure. Daddy, would you and Mom come? Actually, I'd love it if you and Ed and Marcy could all come, but I know that might not be possible with such short notice." Still, Sandy had to swallow, the tears were very close.

"I don't know, my dear. I can surely get the time off, you know that, but I'd hate for your mom to be the one to tell the minister that she has an objection."

Sandy chuckled at that. "That would be something!"

Wishing the best for his firstborn, Charlie said, "My dear, work on your plans and get a date and I'll work on your mom and get this couple in accord. Say, could you introduce me?"

Sandy chuckled. "Of course, Daddy! Daddy, this is Ramon DeLord, Honey, meet my dear daddy, Charlie Bernard."

A deep voice said, "I'm happy to meet you, Mr. Bernard. I also heard your wife, so tell her I'm happy to meet her, too. I really do hope and pray you can convince her that I love your daughter and want only the best for her."

"Young man, I'm pleased to meet you, too. I'm sure we'll have this ironed out before your wedding day."

In the background both Sandy and Ramon heard, "No! It won't ever be worked out! Sandy must come home! I won't allow her to marry, ever!"

"Why, Daddy?"

"The bottom line is, Sandy, your mom can't get beyond your chair."

Through a hiccough, Sandy whispered, "I was afraid of that, Daddy."

* * * * * * * * *

The sun was bright, the air crisp. In the higher elevations of northern Georgia it was definitely fall. Isabel's cabins were booked there would be several extra people in town for the happening taking place on Saturday. Even with the opposition from their mothers, Sandy and Ramon were getting married at ten o'clock in the Blairsville Bible Church. Those that knew the couple were extremely happy for them. Isabel and some of her friends were planning on serving the rehearsal dinner for the families, even though Millie was refusing to come. She was deeply opposed and let everyone know her feelings.

After Ramon had recovered from his meeting with the rock on the trail back in September, he and Duncan had worked out a schedule for the rest of the hiking groups until the end of October, when they would officially close down operations. Duncan had agreed to take the last two groups, so that allowed Sandy and Ramon to set the date for the third Saturday of October. That was tomorrow and Sandy's smile couldn't have been broader. Ramon's grin creased his face, his eyes flashed under his dark eyebrows. Ramon could hardly remember what his life had been like before one lovely, vivacious, Christian lady came to town.

Duncan now lived in Isabel's number two cabin it was smaller than number one, but a man with two good legs had no trouble getting around in it. However, after tomorrow her largest cabin would be empty. She was sorry to see her nearest neighbor moving out, but she was so happy for her and also for Ramon. Ramon on two levels, he was a good man and deserved a good wife, but better than that, he had turned his life over to her Savior. If his mother didn't approve, it was her loss.

Soon after his hospitalization, Ramon remembered his dream that he'd had a few weeks after Sandy arrived. At that time he'd puzzled over the changes he'd visualized happening to his house. Now he'd decided it was a premonition of what he should do. Sandy needed a place in the dry to park her van, especially now that bad weather was only weeks away, so his office was being transformed into a garage. The small bedroom next to the new garage would be the office and Ramon had plans drawn up to add a large master suite onto the back of the house where his weed patch had been during the summer.

When the couple had decided on the date, Sandy painted some announcements, which they sent to their few mutual friends and their families. Much to Sandy's surprise, not only the four people who lived at her home were coming, but also her aunts and uncles who lived north of Philadelphia. She knew they loved her, but she was surprised they could get away from their dairy farm for nearly a week. They were all staying in Isabel's cabins for several nights.

They all planned on arriving Friday afternoon and Sandy was on pins and needles waiting to see her family. She never expected that her dad could talk her mom into coming for her wedding. The scene when she'd left home was still vivid in her mind and probably would be for a long time to come.

Even so, she feared if the minister asked if there were any objections her mom would be the first to jump to her feet, especially since her dad was walking her down the aisle and wouldn't be next to Colleen to keep her quiet. She wondered if that part of the service was really necessary, especially since she wasn't convinced that Millie wouldn't be the second one on her feet to protest the same happening. At first, she'd wanted the wedding at the little church where she'd played her concert, but when she enquired, there was no one in Vansville who could play the wedding march except herself and she wasn't about to play all the music for her own wedding! The organist at the church she, Ramon and Isabel went to in Blairsville had consented to play for them, so that was why they'd planned the wedding for that church.

Everyone involved in the wedding wanted to be sure to have a rehearsal and that was scheduled for Friday evening after a lovely dinner prepared by some of Isabel's friends who lived close by in Vansville. Sandy was glad the little town wasn't far from Blairsville, she was sure at least two of her uncles didn't like to drive at night. The ladies were cooking their food at home, but bringing it to the church on the corner in Vansville where Sandy had performed her concert. Roger had volunteered to set up tables and chairs for the occasion. It would be a festive time, that is, if the mothers let it happen.

Sandy and Ramon sat on the porch of her cabin Friday afternoon as the sun headed for the horizon. Ramon had pulled one of the large living room chairs onto the porch, but before he sat in it, he'd lifted Sandy from her chair and brought her with him to the chair. He loved holding her on his lap and she felt surrounded by his love.

Three cars pulled onto the gravel parking lot. Sandy's face glowed, as she said, "Honey! That's Daddy and Mom, Ed and Marcy in front. The other two cars have two aunts and uncles in each one. They all came!" She touched his face and grinned at him. "You'd better put me back in my chair. Mom's body may be here, but I'm sure she's far from happy."

Ramon chuckled. "I'll do that right away. Besides, you'll want to be closer to them to greet them, I'm sure."

The minute the cars stopped the doors flew open and everyone started talking before they reached Sandy's porch. Ramon carefully lowered Sandy into her chair and she clapped her hands. "I want you to meet my wonderful fiancé, this is Ramon DeLord. Honey, these are dad and mom, Charlie and Colleen Bernard, my brother and sister, Ed and Marcy. These are my aunts and uncles, but we won't worry about names, I know you'll never remember them."

The handsome young man looked at all the people and smiled. "I'm happy to meet you all. Welcome to Vansville, Georgia. We have about an hour before we must be at the church for dinner. The lady who owns these cabins is working with her friends making that dinner, so she's given us the keys for your cabins. We'll take the walk and I'll take you to the door."

"That'll be fine," Charlie said.

Charlie stepped up and as Sandy, with Ramon right beside her came off the porch he hugged her and kissed her cheek. "My dear girl, I've never seen you so happy." He raised his eyes, held out his hand and smiled at her fiancé. "It's nice to meet you in person, Ramon. Welcome to our family."

"Thank you, Sir. I hope I do it justice."

Sandy looked at her mom, she was not smiling or talking and she held her purse in both hands. That told Sandy she had no intentions of shaking Ramon's hand. Sandy smiled at her mom and said, "I'm so glad you came, Mom."

Colleen bent over and kissed her daughter. In her ear, she whispered, "Sandy, there's still time to pack your bags and come home."

Sandy couldn't help it she threw her head back and laughed. "You're funny, Mom! You know that's not going to happen."

Everyone followed Sandy and Ramon down the walk to the other cabins. Ramon let the Bernard's into the first one then opened the next two cabins for the four aunts and uncles. With each one, he said, "We're to meet at the church on the corner at six o'clock for dinner. We'll go from there to the church in Blairsville for the rehearsal."

Charlie had his arm around his wife, but before she could say anything, he said, "That's fine, Ramon, we've been on the road all day and we're glad to stretch our legs. I'm sure the sisters and Marcy want to 'freshen up,' as they say, so we'll meet you here at our cars at six?"

"Make it ten till and that'll be great, Charlie."

"It's as good as done!"

The next morning, Sandy was up with the sun. She still had some packing to do and Ramon was coming with his truck to take everything, including her piano, to his house at seven thirty. They ate a quick breakfast, then Duncan, Roger and Isabel's handyman joined them to move the piano and all of the things Sandy was moving to Ramon's house. The other large thing that needed to be moved was a draped canvas that Sandy had started for Millie's great room. She had it covered Millie hadn't seen it yet, so Sandy wouldn't let anyone see what she'd done.

At nine thirty, Sandy and Marcy were together in the room for the bride. Millie refused to join them and Colleen had insisted that she would dress at the cabin and wait in the foyer to be ushered in. Sandy was disappointed, but she refused to cry on her wedding day. Sandy had picked out a lovely pattern and Isabel had insisted on sewing her wedding dress. Marcy had bought her maid-of-honor dress in Philadelphia. Sandy had no one else to stand with her. Ramon asked Roger to be his best man, but Duncan performed the job of being the usher. All three men were resplendent in their tuxes.

Millie's makeup was flawless, but she held a tissue tightly in her hand and dabbed at her eyes frequently, even as Duncan ushered her and Derek down the aisle. He returned to the back and went to Colleen, but Ed had to bring her to her feet, she wouldn't stand up by herself. Ed shook his head he wanted to spank his childish mother. They followed as Duncan led them down the aisle.

The organist started the Wedding March and the pastor, Ramon and Roger walked in from the side door, while Marcy left the foyer and started down the center aisle. When they were all in place, Sandy and Charlie moved to the center of the doorway. Ed saw them and put his arm under his mom's elbow and raised her to her feet. Everyone else stood up.

Ramon had warned the minister about Colleen and her antagonism and Millie and her dislike of Sandy, so to Colleen's and Millie's surprise, the minister never asked if there was anyone opposed to this union. His first question was, "Who gives this woman to be married to this man?"

Charlie said, "I do."

Tears were streaming down Colleen's face. She was so choked up, her voice was inaudible, as she mouthed the words, "No, no, no! She can't marry him."

"Yes, Mom, she can. Ramon won't let her chair come between them," Ed answered.

CPSIA information can be obtained
at www.ICGtesting.com
Printed in the USA
BVHW081341231020
591516BV00002B/155